Rapid Response Guide
to Opioid Emergencies

Rapid Response Guide to Opioid Emergencies

Greg Clarkes,
ACP, NRP

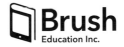

Brush Education Inc.
www.brusheducation.ca
contact@brusheducation.ca

Cover and interior design: Carol Dragich, Dragich Design.
Cover image: Nicola Eddy, Penkee Productions. Images:
water bottle: Ruslan Grumble / Shutterstock.com; Purell hand
sanitizer: BrandonKlein Video / Shutterstock.com; Evzio
auto-injector: AP Photo/Richmond Times-Dispatch, Bob
Brown; all other images: Nicola Eddy, Penkee Productions

Library and Archives Canada Cataloguing in Publication

Title: Rapid response guide to opioid emergencies /
Greg Clarkes, ACP, NRP.

Names: Clarkes, Greg, 1965- author.

Description: Includes bibliographical references.

Identifiers: Canadiana (print) 2020024129X | Canadiana
(ebook) 20200241478 | ISBN 9781550598414 (softcover) |
ISBN 9781550598421 (PDF) | ISBN 9781550598438 (Kindle) |
ISBN 9781550598445 (EPUB)

Subjects: LCSH: Opioid abuse. | LCSH: Opioid abuse—
Treatment. | LCSH: Opioids—Overdose.

Classification: LCC RC568.O45 C53 2020 |
DDC 616.86/3206—dc23

We acknowledge the support of the Government of Canada
Nous reconnaissons l'appui du gouvernement du Canada

Canadä

Contributing reviewers

Claudia Martin, DDS
Director, Postgraduate General Residency Program,
Dentistry Department, Faculty of Medicine and Dentistry,
University of Alberta
Clinical associate, University of Alberta Dental Clinic
Alberta, Canada

Michelle Meyer, PMHNP-B, FNP-BC, MSN
Ohio, USA

Chris Nichol, MD, CCFP
Family physician
Alberta, Canada

JoAnne Seglie, RN, COHN (C)
Occupational health nurse
Workforce Safety and Employee Health, Employee Services
Department,
City of Edmonton
Alberta, Canada

Judy Vandenberg
Advanced care paramedic, Alberta Health Services
Alberta, Canada

Contents

Who should use this guide? viii

1 Equipping yourself for
   opioid emergencies 1

2 How to recognize an opioid
   emergency 37

3 Responding to opioid
   emergencies 42

4 Complications in opioid
   emergencies 73

5 Mixed overdoses: opioids
   with other drugs 79

6 Opioid emergency cases 101

7 A primer on opioids, opioid
   use, and addiction 111

   Abbreviations 124

   About the author 125

Who should use this guide?

This guide is for everyone.

In the current opioid epidemic, opioid emergencies can arise without warning, in situations we didn't anticipate and among those we didn't expect to be affected.

If you are prepared, you can save lives.

You may be a member of the public. Maybe you are a coach, a teacher, a student, a worker in the hospitality industry, the safety officer in your sports club, or a family member of someone who uses prescription opioids or illicit drugs. Generally, you do not have the equipment or training to respond to opioid emergencies. This guide shows you how to prepare and what to do.

You may be a police, security, or corrections officer. You are often first on the scene of opioid emergencies. Some officers have on-the-job equipment and training for responding to opioid emergencies, including emergencies among coworkers from accidental opioid exposure. Many, however, do not. This guide shows you how to prepare and what to do.

You may be a community outreach worker. Community outreach workers are often experienced rescuers, with the knowledge and equipment to respond to opioid emergencies. This guide provides useful review for you. It also discusses possible gaps in safety protocols, and situations that pose particular risks to your personal safety from opioid exposure.

You may be a health-care provider in a hospital or in emergency services. You may be an emergency-room doctor, a unit nurse, or other medical staff in a hospital. Or you may be an emergency medical technician (EMT), a paramedic, a firefighter, or a police officer (depending on the training police receive in your jurisdiction). You are among the best prepared and best trained to respond to opioid emergencies. For you, this guide provides useful review. It also alerts you to situations that pose particular risks to your personal safety from opioid exposure.

You may be a health-care provider in a medical outpatient facility. Outpatient facilities provide dental, orthopedic, and eye surgeries, and other medical procedures. Any medical staff trained to administer opioids in caring for patients (e.g., for sedation or pain) is also trained and equipped to respond to opioid emergencies. For you, this guide provides useful review. For nonmedical assistants in your workplace, it provides crucial information.

You may work at a medical clinic in the community. Maybe you are a doctor, a nurse, or other staff in a medical office or walk-in clinic. Community medical clinics should be prepared for opioid emergencies, which can involve people in crisis brought in by friends or family. Many community medical clinics are not prepared. This guide provides the information you need.

You may be a home-care worker. Home-care workers who provide services to cancer or palliative patients may encounter opioid overdoses because of the pain medications their patients receive. Use this guide to make sure you have what you need and know what to do.

COVID-19 and this guide

The World Health Organization declared COVID-19 a pandemic on March 11, 2020. COVID-19 could continue as a serious public health threat until March 2022. As long as the threat lasts, everyone needs to take steps to protect themselves and to limit the transmission of the virus, including during response to opioid emergencies. Look for alerts like these in this guide: they provide specific advice on responding to opioid emergencies during the COVID-19 pandemic.

Disclaimer

The publisher, authors, contributors, and editors bring substantial expertise to this reference and have made their best efforts to ensure that it is useful, accurate, safe, and reliable.

Nonetheless, practitioners must always rely on their own experience, knowledge and judgment when consulting any of the information contained in this reference or employing it in patient care. When using any of this information, they should remain conscious of their responsibility for their own safety and the safety of others, and for the best interests of those in their care.

To the fullest extent of the law, neither the publishers, the authors, the contributors nor the editors assume any liability for injury or damage to persons or property from any use of information or ideas contained in this reference.

1

Equipping yourself for opioid emergencies

To respond to opioid emergencies, you need:

- personal protective equipment (PPE)
- naloxone

In general, guidelines on PPE and naloxone apply to all types of rescuers.

Where guidelines differ for types of rescuers, this guide offers specific protocols.

A note about CPR training

Training in cardiopulmonary resuscitation (CPR) is part of equipping yourself for opioid emergencies.

This guide assumes that you have at least basic CPR training, which means you already know how to:

- scan a scene for safety, and the person in crisis for injuries
- assess the person for potential spinal injury

- assess level of consciousness, airway, breathing, and circulation, and respond appropriately
- provide ventilation assistance using a face shield or pocket mask with 1-way valve and mucus filter
  - › You may also have training in providing ventilation assistance with bag valve masks, but this is generally beyond basic CPR training. If your job routinely involves responding to opioid emergencies, consider a higher level of CPR training, such as a health-care level, that covers the use of bag valve masks.
- provide compressions when no pulse or signs of circulation are detected
- direct bystanders to help with scene control, call emergency medical services (EMS: 911), and assist with compressions if trained and willing to do so
- place an unconscious person in the recovery position

Because it assumes you have this knowledge, this guide does not go into details about these procedures.

CPR training is mandatory for almost all health-care providers and first responders. It is a good idea for everyone, and is essential in responding to opioid emergencies.

Although it assumes you have basic CPR training, this guide *recommends* better-than-basic training. Better-than-basic training provides instruction in bag valve masks and automatic external defibrillators

(AEDs), and in resuscitation of children and infants (in addition to adults).

CPR courses are available across North America through many agencies. Basic training generally takes 4 to 6 hours and costs less than $100. Higher levels of training, depending on the course, involve slightly more time and cost.

Personal protective equipment (PPE)

Gloves

You need at least 4 pairs of nitrile examination gloves in each size, from small to extra large, in your rapid response equipment. This is because you may tear or damage gloves at the scene of an emergency, or you may have extra helpers on scene. All rescuers at the scene of an emergency need to "double glove" (wear 2 pairs of gloves) with gloves that fit their hands.

Nitrile gloves are recommended over latex gloves. Unlike latex, nitrile does not break down in the presence of fentanyl and carfentanil, which are highly potent and very common synthetic opioids involved in the current opioid crisis. In addition, latex allergies and anaphylaxis are always a concern for both the rescuer and the person in crisis.

If you work in law enforcement, corrections, or security, you may already wear needle-resistant or frisk-type, leather/synthetic gloves. It is acceptable to wear 1 pair of

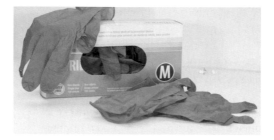

Nitrile gloves: Nitrile gloves generally come all the same size in a box. Ideally, your equipment has a box of each size (S, M, L, XL), or at least 4 pairs of each size in separate, marked, resealable bags.

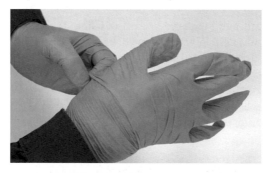

Double gloving: Double gloving means wearing 2 pairs of nitrile gloves.

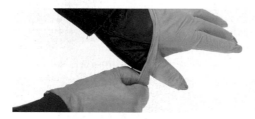

Double gloving with frisk-type gloves: If you wear frisk-type or needle-resistant gloves for your job, and they are in good condition, you can double glove by pulling a pair of nitrile gloves over these gloves.

nitrile gloves over your issued frisk-type or needle-resistant gloves, as long as your issued gloves are in good condition.

Eye protection

You need at least 2 pairs of safety glasses (with side protection, such as side shields) or 2 eye shields in your rapid response equipment. Eye shields are disposable clear lenses that are often attached to disposable face masks, such as dentists and other health-care providers sometimes use.

Appropriate safety glasses and eye shields prevent blood and body fluids, liquids, chemicals, and powders from entering your eyes.

Regular eyeglasses are not as effective as safety glasses, but are better than nothing if, for some reason, safety glasses are not available. It is always better to wear safety glasses or an eye shield over your regular eyeglasses.

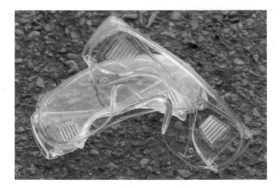

Safety glasses: These come from a variety of manufacturers. Include at least 2 pairs in your equipment.

Respiratory protection

You need at least 2 N95 disposable particulate respirators (masks). N95 particulate respirators provide the minimum protection you need. If you work in health care, or as a first responder, you may have access to more specialized respiratory protection.

Ideally, you should wear respiratory protection at all times when responding to an opioid emergency, because the emergency may involve powdered forms of opioids. If you inhale particles of opioids into your nose, mouth, or respiratory tract, you—the rescuer—may absorb them and become a second victim of the opioid.

This means you should use a bag valve mask to provide artificial ventilations to a person in crisis, if you have the required training: a bag valve mask allows you to keep your respiratory protection on while caring for the person in crisis.

If your job requires you to wear any type of respirator, occupational standards and regulations require you to be fit tested. Fit testing ensures respirators fit your face properly. The National Institute for Occupational Safety and Health (NIOSH) in the United States requires fit testing at least annually, and the Canadian Standards Association (CSA) requires fit testing every 2 years.

If your job gives you access to specialized respiratory protection, you can use it instead of an N95 particulate respirator. For example, dangerous goods teams have full-face respirators with cartridge-type filters

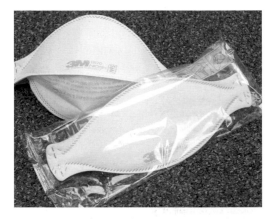

N95 particulate respirators: These come from several manufacturers in boxes of 20 or more. Include at least 2 respirators in your equipment. Note that the "flat fold" type of respirator (e.g., the 3M 1870+ Aura Health Care Particulate Respirator) can be stored or carried flat, which suits it for opioid-response PPE. If your role as a rescuer involves frequent exposure to blood or body fluids, choose a fluid-resistant N95 particulate respirator.

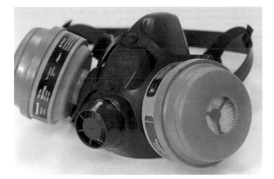

Half-mask respirator: If you have access to specialized respiratory protection through your job, such as this half-mask cartridge respirator, use it instead of an N95 particulate respirator.

(these include eye protection), and firefighters have self-contained breathing apparatus (SCBA). Make sure you are properly fit tested for this equipment.

If you do not regularly wear respirators for your job, make sure you know and practice the procedures for putting on and taking off the N95 particulate respirators in your PPE. Manufacturers of N95 particulate respirators provide detailed instructions on these procedures, which protect you from contamination and are essential to your safety.

COVID-19 and PPE

In treating people with possible COVID-19, public health agencies identify procedures that generate droplets as a particular risk to those providing care.[1,2] Cardiopulmonary resuscitation is considered a procedure that generates droplets[1,3] and it is often an essential procedure in responding to opioid emergencies.

The PPE that protects rescuers from accidental exposure to opioids also protects them from droplets, **except** that current guidelines also recommend gowns. The complete list of minimum recommended PPE is:[1,2]

- nitrile gloves (opioid emergencies require double gloving, which is more protection than required for droplet protection)
- safety glasses or eye shield (prescription eye glasses **are not** considered adequate protection)
- fit-tested N95 particulate respirator, or higher-level respirator
- gown

Stay up to date. Check online for updates from public health agencies in your jurisdiction for the latest recommendations on PPE during the pandemic. Also keep up to date on routine vaccines and specialized vaccines that may arise as this, and other viruses or bacteria, emerge and evolve.

Protection for providing ventilation assistance

There are 2 ways to provide ventilation assistance to a person in crisis:

- via a bag valve mask
- via a pocket mask with a 1-way valve and, ideally, a mucus filter

Bag valve masks require training, which is generally not a standard part of basic CPR courses, although some instructors include it in basic courses anyway. Bag valve masks are an advantage in responding to opioid

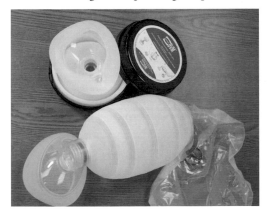

Compressible bag valve mask: This type of bag valve mask fits into a small case, which makes it space efficient and very portable. This image shows 2 of these masks: 1 packed into its black circular case (top of image), and 1 fully deployed (bottom of image).

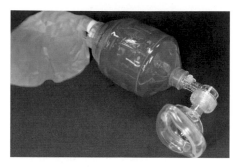

Bag valve mask: This type of bag valve mask is not compressible. It is the kind generally used in hospitals and in emergency services.

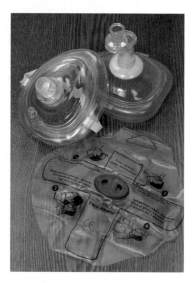

Pocket masks: This image shows 3 types of pocket masks. Two of them (bottom and upper left) have 1-way valves. The mask in the upper-right corner also has a mucus filter. Pocket masks come from a variety of manufacturers in boxes that contain 1 or several masks. Include at least 2 in your equipment (unless you have a bag valve mask and are trained to use it).

emergencies because they allow you to keep your respiratory protection on while caring for a person in crisis. Without a bag valve mask, you must remove your respiratory protection to give artificial respiration. Removing your respiratory protection exposes you to the risk of inhaling particles of opioids, which could incapacitate you and even result in overdose.

If you have training in the use of bag valve masks, include at least 1 bag valve mask in your equipment.

If you do not have training in the use of bag valve masks, include at least 2 pocket masks with a 1-way valve and, ideally, a mucus filter in your equipment. Some first-aid pocket masks have a 1-way valve, but no mucus filter. Mucus filters prevent liquids and particulates from entering the valve and provide increased protection from biohazards to the rescuer providing ventilations.

Only use a pocket mask when safe to do so. Any visible powder on the person in crisis or at the scene means it is best *not* to remove your respiratory protection. Note, however, that you can reduce risks from on-scene powders by thoroughly flushing them with water.

COVID-19 and equipment for ventilation assistance

If you work in emergency services, note that the Centers for Disease Control and Prevention recommend high-efficiency particulate air (HEPA) filters for expired air from bag valve masks.[1]

If you are any other kind of rescuer, consider providing hands-only CPR during the pandemic, as

recommended by some agencies.[4] **This recommendation means you should not provide ventilation
assistance via any kind of pocket mask** unless the
COVID-19 status of the person in crisis is known
to you. For example, the person in crisis may be
a family member whom you know is negative for
the virus.

Stay up to date. Check online for updates from
public health agencies in your jurisdiction for the
latest recommendations on providing ventilation
assistance during the pandemic.

Hand sanitizer

Include a small pocket-sized bottle of hand
sanitizer in your equipment. However, avoid
alcohol-based hand sanitizers: these accelerate
the absorption of synthetic opioids, such as
fentanyl and carfentanil, that may end up on
your skin.

Note that it is important to decontaminate
with soap and water as soon as possible if

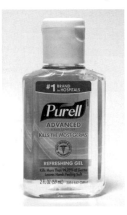

Hand sanitizer: Choose a non-alcohol-based hand
sanitizer from among the many brands available.

powdered or liquid opioids may be on your skin. Avoid washing with hypochlorite bleach solutions: these, like alcohol-based hand sanitizers, may accelerate absorption of synthetic opioids.

Bottled water

Consider including 1 or 2 bottles of drinking water, depending on the space you have available in your rapid response equipment. You can use water to flush powders on or near a person in crisis, which reduces your risk inhaling opioids. You can also use it for primary decontamination of yourself, to flush your eyes or skin, as needed.

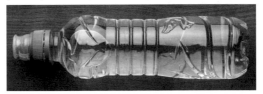

Bottled drinking water: Space restrictions in storing your PPE may determine whether you can include a bottle of water. You can use water to flush powders at the scene of an emergency, or to flush your eyes or skin, as needed.

Naloxone

Naloxone can be administered in several ways. The delivery system you use depends on your source of naloxone.

If you are a health-care provider in a hospital, an outpatient clinic, or emergency services, you will be working with naloxone-delivery systems supplied through your job and for which you are trained.

If you are any other kind of rescuer, you will likely be working with naloxone supplied in a ready-made kit, or in a kit you assemble yourself. The information about naloxone that follows is mostly for you.

Make sure you know the naloxone-delivery system you are working with. Make sure you have adequate training and practice to use it. **If you do not have specific training in using naloxone through your job,** try to acquire practice supplies from a pharmacy, CPR instructor, or community agency.

How naloxone counteracts opioids

Opioids circulating in the blood attach to opioid receptors in the body, primarily in the brain and spinal cord. Naloxone, which was created to reverse the effects of opioids, also attaches to opioid receptors. It fights for these receptors: it removes opioids from receptors and then takes their place. It's like removing someone from a chair and then sitting in the chair yourself.

Naloxone is very effective at displacing opioids from receptors, but it does not have staying power. It is effective for only 5 to 30 minutes, on average.

Opioids displaced from receptors by naloxone reenter the bloodstream. They can reattach to opioid receptors when the naloxone is no longer effective. Unlike the short 5-to-30-minute lifespan of naloxone, opioids may last in the body for hours.

This means that a person in crisis may revive after administration of naloxone, and then fall back into unconsciousness. Repeat doses of naloxone may be needed to save their life.

Naloxone can be administered by intravenous (IV), intranasal (IN), or intramuscular (IM) routes. Of these routes, IN injection (intranasal spray) is the simplest. Nasal spray absorbs into the tissues of the nasal cavity, and it is as effective as IV or IM routes in reversing opioid overdose.[5,6] In addition, a 2013 study suggests that addicts, who can become aggressive when treated with naloxone, may be less aggressive when treated with nasal spray because they return to consciousness more gradually.[6]

Ready-made naloxone kits

You can buy ready-made naloxone kits at some pharmacies and online. In many parts of North America, governments provide naloxone kits for free. Types of ready-made kits include:

- Narcan nasal spray, which is a type of intranasal (IN) injection system
- other IN injection systems
- intramuscular (IM) injection systems

Check that the kit has adequate amounts of naloxone. The doses in some ready-made kits were established before synthetic opioids, such as fentanyl and carfentanil, became common as illicit drugs: the kits may not contain enough total naloxone to reverse overdoses from these drugs. Some overdoses involving synthetic opioids require a total of 8 mg to 16 mg of naloxone (and occasionally more) to reverse.

If your kit does not contain adequate naloxone, consider supplementing it with naloxone you buy at a pharmacy or online, or consider making your own kit. Note that if you supplement naloxone in any needle-based kit, you need to include at least 1 more syringe and needle for each added dose.

Narcan nasal spray

Narcan nasal spray is the most effective, the most rapid, and the safest way to deliver naloxone. It comes in ready-to-use 4-mg dispensers. Each dispenser delivers a 4-mg dose.

To use Narcan nasal spray:

1. **Put on your PPE.**

2. **Hold the dispenser with your fingers on either side of the nozzle and your thumb on the plunger.**

3. **Direct the nozzle up a nostril of the person in crisis.** Ideally, the person is on their back with their head tilted back.

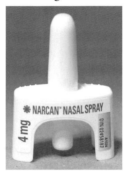

Narcan nasal spray dispenser: This is a self-contained and ready-to-use device, with a nozzle and a preloaded dose of naloxone.

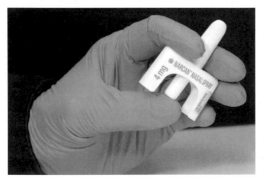

Holding position for Narcan nasal spray: Put your fingers on either side of the nozzle and your thumb on the plunger.

4. **Quickly push the plunger as far as it will go.** You may feel resistance and a small click when the plunger has fully discharged the naloxone.

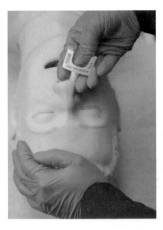

Narcan nasal spray administration: Direct the nozzle up a nostril of the person in crisis and push the plunger as far as it will go.

Other intranasal (IN) injection kits

Other IN injection kits may contain ready-to-use dispensers. Many, however, are "preload syringe" systems with items that you need to assemble: separate ampoules of naloxone, syringe barrels that accept the ampoules, and mucosal atomization devices ("nasal tips").

These kits are different from Narcan nasal spray. The preloaded doses in the dispensers or ampoules are not as large (the doses are typically 2 mg, as opposed to 4 mg with Narcan nasal spray), which means you may need to administer more doses to a person in crisis than with Narcan nasal spray.

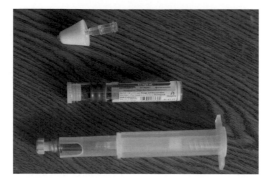

IN injection preload-syringe system: This system has syringe barrels, preloaded ampoules of naloxone that screw into the syringe barrels, and nasal tips that screw onto the top of the syringe barrels.

In addition, if they contain items that need assembly, they are not as convenient or as fast to use.

IN injection kits may also contain 1 pair of nitrile gloves (size large) and a disposable CPR face shield. You should supplement and customize this PPE, following the PPE guidelines at the beginning of this chapter.

To administer an IN injection from a ready-made preload-syringe kit:

1. **Put on your PPE.**

2. **Screw the ampoule into the syringe barrel.** You need to remove the covers from the top of the ampoule and the bottom of the syringe barrel first.

3. **Screw the nasal tip onto the syringe barrel.** Remove the top of the syringe barrel first. The nasal tip is not sterile: it's okay to touch it with your gloved hands.

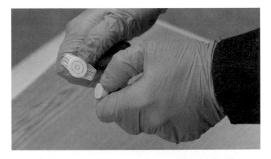

Opening the bottom of the syringe barrel and top of the ampoule: Pop off the covers with your thumbs.

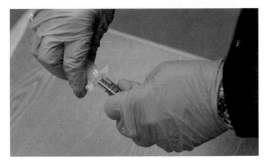

Screwing in the ampoule: Insert the ampoule into the syringe barrel and screw it into place.

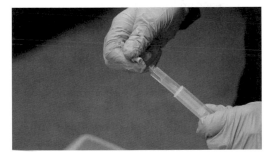

Opening the top of the syringe barrel: Twist the cover and pull it off.

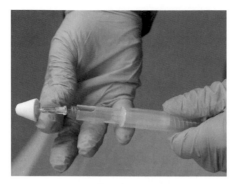

Screwing on the nasal tip: Use your gloved hands to do this (the nasal tip isn't sterile).

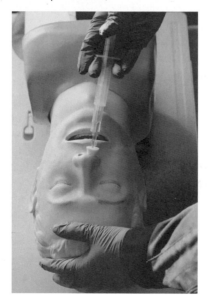

Administering naloxone via the nasal tip: Direct the nasal tip up a nostril of the person in crisis and push the bottom of the ampoule as far as it will go.

4. **Direct the nasal tip up a nostril of the person in crisis** . Ideally, the person is on their back with their head tilted back.

5. **Quickly push the bottom of the ampoule as far as it will go.**

Intramuscular (IM) injection kits

Some IM injection kits are Evzio auto-injectors. These are devices that inject a preloaded 2-mg dose of naloxone when you press the device against the thigh of a person in crisis. They provide the easiest way of injecting naloxone (they can inject through clothing), and also have safety features to protect rescuers from needlestick injuries.

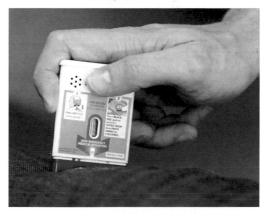

Evzio auto-injector: This is a self-contained IM injection system with a preloaded 2-mg dose of naloxone. It is the easiest IM injection system to use. Note that the demonstrator is missing nitrile gloves in this photograph, but rescuers should always wear full PPE when using the Evzio auto-injector (or any naloxone-delivery system) in a real situation.

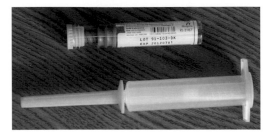

IM injection preload-syringe system: This system has syringe barrels (with needles attached) and ampoules of naloxone that screw into the syringe barrels. In this example, the needle is inside a cover.

Some IM injection kits are preload-syringe systems, where (as with preload-syringe systems for IN injection) you screw ampoules of naloxone into syringe barrels. The syringe barrels typically have needles attached.

Many IM injection kits are "manual draw" systems, where you draw the naloxone through a needle into a syringe from an ampoule. This system is the most complicated way of delivering naloxone.

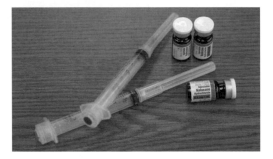

IM injection manual-draw system: This system has syringes (with needles attached) and ampoules of naloxone. You draw the naloxone into the syringe via the needle.

Using needle-based systems requires training, practice, and a cool head. Panic and fear in an emergency situation can result in mistakes, loss of medication, and possible needlestick injury to you, the rescuer. As well, unless you are working with an auto-injector, it always takes longer to administer naloxone by injection than by Narcan nasal spray. This means more time spent on supportive care such as ventilations or compressions.

If you are working with a needle-based system, check whether the syringes are "safety syringes" (technically known as "safety engineered sharps").

Safety syringes are a great asset in health care, because they prevent needlestick injuries. However, they require more training and practice to operate effectively than nonsafety syringes and needles. Naloxone kits for the public often contain safety syringes. In safety syringes, the needle automatically retracts into the barrel of the syringe after the plunger of the syringe is fully depressed. Because of this safety feature, these syringes come from the manufacturer with plungers that are not fully depressed, and they are meant to be filled by pulling back the plunger from this initial position. First-aiders and non-health-care workers in a panic situation often think they need to expel air from a newly opened safety syringe before filling it. They may press the plunger all the way into the syringe and trigger the needle to automatically retract, which renders the entire syringe and needle useless. **If your kit has safety syringes,** make sure you carry

several spares, in case you make mistakes with
them during an emergency. It's also useful to
practice using them regularly, so you make
fewer mistakes.

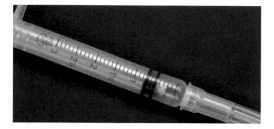

Plunger position in a newly opened safety syringe: In
a newly opened safety syringe, like this one, the plunger
is not fully depressed. Do not make the mistake of
depressing the plunger before filling the syringe. If you
push the plunger as far as it will go, you will trigger the
automatic retraction of the needle (its safety feature)
and render the entire syringe useless.

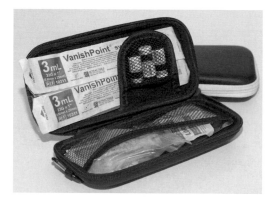

Ready-made manual-draw kit with safety syringes:
This free naloxone kit contains VanishPoint syringes, a
type of safety syringe. Safety syringes are common in
kits available for free.

Note that IM injection kits often contain alcohol wipes for the injection site, 1 pair of nitrile gloves (size large), and a disposable CPR face shield. You should supplement and customize this PPE, following the PPE guidelines at the beginning of this chapter.

To administer an IM injection from a ready-made manual-draw kit:

1. **Put on your PPE.**

2. **Open the syringe-and-needle package from the plunger end.** This keeps the needle as clean as possible.

3. **Open the top of the naloxone ampoule.** Pop off the protective tip.

4. **Note the silicone seal on the ampoule: keep it sterile.** The silicone seal is at the center of the top of the ampoule. Do not touch this with your hands.

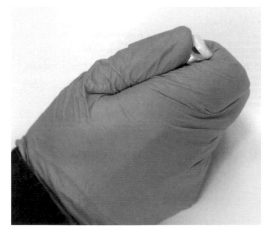

Opening a naloxone ampoule: Pop off the protective tip of the ampoule with your thumb.

5. **Remove the cover from the needle**. Be careful! Put the cover down on a clean surface, because you will need to recap the needle.

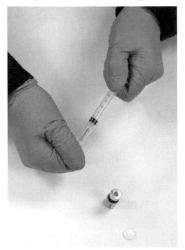

Removing a needle cover: Be careful not to stick yourself.

6. **Direct the needle into the ampoule through the silicone seal.** Push it to the bottom of the ampoule.

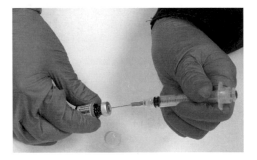

Directing a needle into an ampoule: Push the needle through the silicone seal.

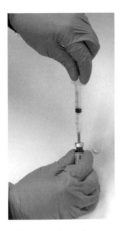 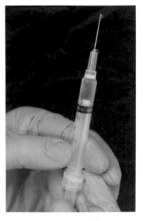

Filling a syringe from an ampoule: Slowly pull back on the plunger.

Expelling air from a syringe: Keep the needle up.

7. **Draw all of the contents of the ampoule into the syringe.** Hold the ampoule at an angle, with the needle at the bottom of the ampoule, and slowly pull back on the plunger of the syringe.

8. **Expel any air in the syringe.** Hold the needle upright (needle up) to do this. Be careful!

9. **Recap the needle.** Be careful! With the cover lying on a surface, scoop the cover with the needle. Then, push the cover and

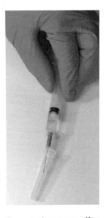

Recapping a needle: Put the cover and the needle on a surface. Scoop the cover with the needle, and push the cover tightly to the syringe.

syringe together. Make sure the cover is tightly secured to the syringe.

10. **Clean the injection site** with an alcohol wipe. The injection site should be the person's arm, thigh, or buttock: choose the most easily accessible site with the greatest amount of muscle tissue.

11. **Remove the cover from the needle.** Be careful!

12. **Inject the naloxone.** Insert the needle into the injection site and push the plunger as far as it will go. If you are working with a safety syringe, make sure you push the plunger until the needle safely retracts into the syringe.

Building your own naloxone kit

You can build your own naloxone kit from scratch, with supplies available at pharmacies and online. In many jurisdictions in North America, pharmacies supply naloxone in all forms without a prescription. In addition, anyone can buy Narcan nasal spray online from its manufacturer, Adapt Pharma.

For Narcan nasal spray, you should include at least 2 dispensers (each with a 4-mg dose, for a total of 8 mg) in the kit you build. The dispensers come in boxes of 2, so you would need at least 1 box.

For all other systems, make sure you have a total of at least 8 mg of naloxone. If the system involves 2-mg doses of naloxone, this means you need to include at least 4 doses. You also need enough equipment to deliver all the doses to a person in crisis.

How much equipment do you need?

- **Preload-syringe systems for IN injection:** You don't need a new nasal tip or syringe barrel to give repeat doses. You screw the next ampoule into the same barrel, with the same nasal tip attached. It's good to have backup equipment, though, so you should include at least 2 syringe barrels and 2 nasal tips in the naloxone kit you build.

- **IM injection systems (preload-syringe and manual-draw):** You need a new needle and syringe for each repeat dose.
  › Generally, you can buy preload-syringe systems for IM injection by the box. Each box contains a 2-mg ampoule of naloxone and a syringe with a needle attached. So, you would need at least 4 boxes in your naloxone kit.

  › Manual-draw systems are generally not prepackaged: you would need to buy syringes and needles separately from the ampoules of naloxone. Ampoules typically have 2 mg of naloxone per 2 mL. So, you would need at least 4 of these. You would also need at least 8 needles (23 to 25 gauge) in 2 lengths: 1.5 inches (2.5 cm) and 1 inch (40 mm). Use shorter needles on people with less muscle tissue.

  › It's easy to make mistakes with manual-draw systems, so consider including spare ampoules, needles, and syringes.

› You can purchase needles, syringes, and alcohol wipes online. In many communities, you can also buy them at home-health-care stores and pharmacies. They generally come in boxes with many needles and syringes (e.g., boxes of 100).

A note about mucosal atomization devices for IM injection systems

You can buy mucosal atomization devices ("nasal tips") for manual-draw systems that have luer-lock syringes. A luer lock allows you to screw attachments onto the syringe, including needles and nasal tips.

The steps for using this type of system follow procedures already described for attaching nasal tips and using manual-draw systems. Consult the images for those procedures for more information. Note that advanced first responders, such as paramedics, are more likely to use this type of system.

To administer an IN injection with a manual-draw system:

1. **Put on your PPE.**

2. **Open the syringe-and-needle package from the plunger end.** This keeps the needle as clean as possible.

3. **Open the top of the naloxone ampoule.** Pop off the protective tip.

4. **Note the silicone seal on the ampoule: keep it sterile.** The silicone seal is at the center of the top of the ampoule. Do not touch this with your hands.

5. **Remove the cover from the needle.** Be careful! Put the cover down on a clean surface. You will need to recap the needle.

6. **Direct the needle into the ampoule through the silicone seal.** Push it to the bottom of the ampoule.

7. **Draw all of the contents of the ampoule into the syringe.** Hold the ampoule at an angle, with the needle at the bottom of the ampoule, and slowly pull back on the plunger of the syringe. Don't worry about air in the syringe.

8. **Recap the needle.** Be careful! With the cover lying on a surface, direct the needle into the cover.

9. **Unscrew the covered needle from the syringe.**

10. **Screw the nasal tip onto the syringe.** The nasal tip is not sterile, so it's okay to touch it with your gloved hands.

11. **Direct the nasal tip up the nostril of the person in crisis.** Ideally, the person is on their back with their head tilted back.

12. **Quickly push the plunger as far as it will go.**

Why should you build your own naloxone kit?

Building your own custom kit may be a good option if the only ready-made kit available to you is needle based. As a first-aid instructor and paramedic, I can tell you that administration of a drug without needles is ideal.

It may also be a good option if you need a kit protected from extremes of weather, dust, or moisture. Consider how the conditions in which you would typically respond to an emergency might make different delivery systems more or less practical, and how they might affect the way you store your naloxone supply.

Always keep PPE on hand with your naloxone kit.

Building a naloxone kit: police, corrections, and security officers

If you work in law enforcement, corrections, or security, you may want to build your own naloxone kit, as well as a personal first-aid kit (PFAK), to ensure that you have the equipment you need as a frontline responder. You are often first on the scene at an opioid crisis: because of this, you are at highest risk among rescuers of exposure to opioids. The kits you build should fit your needs and your mission, and be based on your experience and knowledge of the community you serve.

My minimum equipment recommendations are:

- **PFAK (for you, the rescuer)**
  - › **naloxone kit with PPE,** *carried on you at all times*
    - » 2 to 4 Narcan nasal spray dispensers, for use on you or a buddy
    - » 2 pairs of nitrile gloves that fit your hands
    - » 2 N95 particulate respirators
  - › **other first-aid supplies, carried in a go bag**
    - » several pairs of different-sized nitrile gloves

» several N95 particulate respirators, or individual half-mask respirators (all types of respirators require fit testing)
» eye protection
» 1 or 2 bag valve masks
» 1 or 2 bottles of drinking water for primary decontamination
» tourniquet, for life-threatening blood loss to a limb
» hemostatic gauze, which is a specialized gauze impregnated with clot-promoting substances
» shears, for cutting through uniform clothing or strapping
» thermal barrier to ensure retention of body heat until EMS arrives

- **naloxone kit, PPE, and first-aid supplies for a person in crisis, carried in a go bag**

  › 4 to 8 Narcan nasal spray dispensers (a total of 2 to 4 boxes)
  › several pairs of different-sized nitrile gloves
  › several N95 particulate respirators, or individual half-mask respirators (all types of respirators require fit testing)
  › eye protection
  › 1 or 2 bag valve masks
  › 1 or 2 bottles of drinking water for primary decontamination
  › AED
  › tourniquets, hemostatic dressings, and shears

> › pressure dressing for bleeding not requiring tourniquets or wound packing with hemostatic agent
> › thermal barrier

Storing and maintaining your rapid response equipment

If you are a health-care provider in a hospital or in emergency services, your PPE and naloxone-delivery system are likely checked at regular intervals to ensure all supplies are in place and not expired.

If you are any other kind of rescuer, check your PPE and naloxone-delivery system regularly to ensure all supplies are in place and not expired. Many supplies come stamped with expiry dates (e.g., naloxone, hand sanitizer); for other supplies, look online for the recommendations of the manufacturer. Consider keeping all of your rapid response equipment (PPE and naloxone kit) in a clear plastic container with a small plastic breakaway seal: the plastic container allows you to identify first-aid supplies at a glance; the breakaway seal indicates whether the equipment has been used between checks. In schools, community buildings, and workplaces, consider storing rapid response equipment in a hard-sided case mounted on a wall next to other emergency equipment, such as first-aid kits, AEDs, or fire extinguishers. Put a sign on the case (e.g., "Naloxone") and install signs to indicate its location.

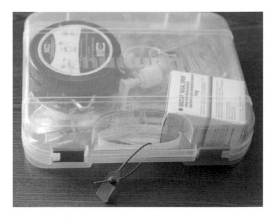

Example of how to store rapid response equipment:
The breakaway seal on this container is intact,
indicating that the equipment is complete and ready
to use. Check rapid response equipment regularly to
ensure it is complete and to replace items that have
expired.

What to do with used PPE and naloxone kits

All used PPE and naloxone-delivery items
are potentially infectious or a chemical risk.
Discard and replace all items used to respond
to an opioid emergency. Note that disposal
procedures vary by jurisdiction. Specific procedures may include special bagging or boxing
for items, and incineration.

The only exception is safety glasses, which
you can carefully wash with soap and water
(double glove with nitrile gloves while doing
this). Wash them twice: once to clean and
once to disinfect. Consider disposing of safety
glasses, however, if they have blood or body
fluids on them.

If you are a health-care provider in a hospital or in emergency services, follow the protocols in place for discarding biohazards, sharps, and used or expired medications.

If you are any other kind of rescuer, you will likely call EMS (911) for assistance. EMS, including ambulances and fire-rescue vehicles, have sharps containers for needles, and appropriate containers for contaminated clothing, equipment, and biohazards.

REFERENCES

1 Centers for Disease Control and Prevention. Interim guidance for emergency medical services (EMS) and 911 public safety answering points (PSAPS) for COVID-19 in the United States [Internet]. [Atlanta (GA)]: CDC; [updated 2020 10 March; cited 2020 15 April]. Available from https://www.cdc.gov/coronavirus/2019-ncov/hcp/guidance-for-ems.html

2 Public Health Agency of Canada. Corona virus (COVID-19): For health professionals [Internet]. [Ottawa (ON)]: The Agency; [updated 2020 April 11; cited 2020 April 15]. Available from https://www.canada.ca/en/public-health/services/diseases/2019-novel-coronavirus-infection/health-professionals.html?topic=tilelink

3 Public Health Ontario. IPAC recommendations for use of personal protective equipment for care of individuals with suspect or confirmed COVID-19 [Internet]. [Toronto (ON)]: Public Health Ontario; [updated 2020 April 6; cited 2020 April 15]. Available from https://www.publichealthontario.ca/-/media/documents/ncov/updated-ipac-measures-covid-19.pdf?la=en

4 Heart and Stroke Foundation of Canada. Modifications to public hands-only CPR during the COVID-19 pandemic [Internet]. Ottawa (ON): The Foundation; [updated 2020 6 April; cited 2020 April 15]. Available from https://www.heartandstroke.ca/articles/modification-to-hands-only-cpr-during-the-covid-19-pandemic

5 World Health Organization. Community management of opioid overdose. Geneva: World Health Organization, 2014. 74 p.

6 Wermeling D. A response to the opioid overdose epidemic: naloxone nasal spray. *Drug Deliv Tranl Res*. 2013;3(1):63–74. doi: 10.1007/s13346-012-0092-0

2

How to recognize an opioid emergency

Signs and symptoms of opioid overdose

All opioid overdoses, including overdoses from synthetic opioids, have similar signs and symptoms.

Commonly taught core triad of symptoms

- **decreased level of consciousness**
  - › This can range from a mild decrease to complete loss of consciousness.

- **decreased respiration**
  - › Breathing slows and becomes shallow (bradypnea). It may become irregular. Symptoms can progress to respiratory arrest, where breathing completely stops (apnea).

- **pinpoint pupils**
  - › This means the pupils are very small.

Other symptoms

- **euphoria**
- **decreased sensations of pain**
- **decreased heart rate and pulse strength**
  - › Decreased heart rate (bradycardia) can lead to poor circulation (shock), and a drop in blood pressure (hypotension). Cardiac arrest is possible with opioid overdose.

- **irregular heartbeat (dysrhythmia)**
  - › This may occur as oxygen reaching the heart muscle decreases.

- **pale, cool, clammy skin**
- **blue coloring around the mouth and on the fingernails**
  - › This may occur as oxygen reaching other parts of the body decreases, and carbon dioxide in the blood increases, making venous blood a darker color.

- **seizures and convulsions**
  - › These may occur.

- **no cough response or gag reflex**
  - › This may present as regurgitation of stomach contents, or as a gurgling noise. Note that the person in crisis risks aspirating (inhaling) stomach contents into the lungs at any stage of a rescue, including when administration of naloxone reverses the effects of opioids.

Other on-scene indicators of opioid overdose

Other on-scene indicators are not as important as the signs and symptoms of overdose, but may still be useful.

Note that *knowing* a crisis is an opioid emergency is not as crucial as acting appropriately *if it is a possibility*.

Note also that *acting appropriately* includes taking steps to ensure your personal safety as a rescuer. Particular risks to you include needles (because you can stick yourself with contaminated needles) and powdered drugs (because you can inhale them).

If you are on the scene of an emergency in the community (e.g., the person in crisis is in a public washroom, on the street, or in their bedroom at home), assess the scene. You may find information that will help the person in crisis and will keep you safe.

See Chapter 3 on responding to opioid emergencies for more on scene assessment.

Consider what you know or can quickly establish about the situation.

- The person may be a friend or family member whom you know takes prescription opioids or recreational drugs.
- Ask bystanders for information: Was the person using drugs? What drugs? Did anyone see the person lose consciousness? What happened?
- Scan the scene for evidence of drugs.
  › Opioids enter the body through 4 routes, possibly in combination: injection

(needles), ingestion (pills or liquids), inhalation (powders), and absorption (transdermal patch, or unintentional fentanyl or carfentanil powder or liquid on the skin).

› In addition, be aware that any way of taking any illicit drug (e.g., cocaine, methamphetamine, phencyclidine) is also a route of exposure to opioids, because any illicit drug can be mixed with powerful synthetic opioids such as fentanyl and carfentanil.

What if you give naloxone to someone *not* in an opioid emergency?

At the scene of an emergency, it may be difficult to determine whether a person in crisis is suffering from an opioid overdose or something else: a variety of conditions can cause decreased levels of conscious.

What if you're not sure?

The rule of thumb is: when in doubt, give naloxone.

The consequences of *not* giving naloxone, if a person *needs* naloxone, are greater than the consequences of giving naloxone to someone who doesn't need it. Naloxone has minimally significant side effects if given when not required. However, a person who needs naloxone because of an opioid overdose may die if they don't get naloxone.

Many conditions may cause symptoms that resemble opioid overdose, such as diabetic emergencies, respiratory and cardiac arrest, stroke, anaphylaxis, hypothermia, shock, and exposure to toxins (e.g., pesticides).

However, in the current opioid crisis, opioid overdose is a major cause of crisis in people found with decreased levels of consciousness, or in respiratory arrest (no breathing) or cardiopulmonary arrest (no breathing and no pulse).

In addition, be aware that opioids can provoke cardiac arrest.

Before the current opioid crisis (before 2015), the majority of cardiac arrests were caused by a condition called sudden cardiac arrest (SCA). SCA is primarily the result of sudden disturbances in the electrical conduction system of the heart. Persons suffering from SCA may or may not have a preexisting cardiac condition, and may be young or old.

In the current opioid crisis, many cardiac arrests directly result from opioid overdose. The World Health Organization recommends health-care providers administer naloxone early in the care of cardiac-arrest patients in cases of suspected opioid overdose.[1] If a person in cardiac arrest has no pulse, naloxone can still help them if the cause is opioid overdose: chest compressions provided through cardiopulmonary resuscitation (CPR) circulate naloxone through the body.

REFERENCES

1 World Health Organization. Community management of opioid overdose. Geneva: World Health Organization, 2014. 74 p.

3

Responding to opioid emergencies

Opioid emergencies fall into 2 categories: they happen in monitored settings, where the circumstances of overdose are known; or in unmonitored settings in the community, where the circumstances of overdose are unknown.

This section mostly focuses on opioid emergencies in unmonitored settings (opioid emergency scenes in the community).

Types of opioid emergencies

Opioid overdoses in monitored settings

Emergencies in monitored settings pose few risks to rescuers of opioid exposure or other injury.

The person in crisis may be a patient in a hospital, receiving opioids as part of their treatment; or an outpatient undergoing procedural sedation for a dental or eye procedure; or a person using drugs at a safe-injection site, where the focus is harm reduction. The rescuer may be a unit nurse, an attending physician, a medical assistant, or a community outreach worker.

In monitored settings, overdose may happen because of an unexpected reaction to a known opioid treatment or drug, or because of synthetic opioids in drugs of abuse. Rescuers know that powdered forms of illicit drugs—a possible threat in other circumstances—are less likely to be an issue (but the possibility should not be dismissed out of hand).

In hospitals and outpatient clinics, opioid overdoses are typically treated by injecting naloxone intravenously. At safe-injection sites, rescuers have naloxone available and are ready to use it.

In monitored settings, the key step in responding to opioid emergencies is to have naloxone available. If you provide sedation or pain medication to patients, make sure you have quick access to naloxone and the training to use it. Keep enough medication on your countertop with enough needles and syringes.

Opioid emergency scenes in the community

Responding to an opioid emergency scene in the community is more complex than responding to an overdose in a monitored setting.

Emergency scenes pose risks of opioid exposure to rescuers. The risks are potentially high. Other risks to personal safety are also possible, depending on the circumstances of the emergency.

Examples of opioid emergency scenes in the community include public washrooms, vehicles, concert venues, and homes. The person in crisis may have collapsed at a party, at work, on the street, or in their bedroom. The reason for their crisis may not be immediately apparent.

From an emergency scene in the community, a person in crisis may be transported to a hospital emergency room (ER). They may come by ambulance, or friends or family may bring them. Friends and family may also take a person in crisis to a community medical clinic or outreach center.

In situations involving opioid emergency scenes in the community, or people from these scenes, personal protection for rescuers is essential. Your well-being as a rescuer allows you to assist the person in crisis, and protects everyone around you.

Responding to an opioid emergency scene in the community: general procedure

Assess the scene
Scene assessment alerts you to hazards to your personal safety.

Hazards at a scene may include extreme weather, poor lighting, potentially dangerous people, traffic, and drug paraphernalia, such

as powder or needles on or near the victim.
Body fluids, such as vomitus or blood-tinged
saliva, may be on or near the victim, and these
may contain pathogens.

Note all hazards and prepare to respond
appropriately.

**If you do not work in emergency ser-
vices,** the situation may be unusual to you,
and the environment may not feel safe to
approach. Listen to your instincts. This does
not mean you cannot be of assistance. If you
decide to withdraw to a safer location, contact
emergency medical services (EMS: 911) and
alert others in the area of your concerns and
suspicions. This assistance alone is significant
in responding to an emergency scene.

Call emergency medical services (EMS: 911)

If you work in emergency services, this
step obviously doesn't apply to you. However,
when you arrive on scene, consider whether
you need additional EMS support, or assistance from a dangerous goods team or law
enforcement.

**If you do not work in emergency ser-
vices,** ask a bystander to call EMS (911), or
call yourself. Set the phone to speaker mode,
and work with EMS dispatchers to provide first aid. In almost every part of North
America, emergency dispatchers provide
information and instructions to assist you
in the care of a person in crisis prior to the
arrival of EMS. These dispatch professionals
follow a script to provide instructions. They

are calm and professional, and a key resource
during an emergency.

Work with a buddy if possible

Working with a buddy allows steps in care to
proceed simultaneously. For example, a buddy
can provide cardiopulmonary resuscitation
(CPR) while you administer naloxone.

A buddy can also rescue you, if you are
exposed to opioids on scene and need help.
All rescuers should stay alert to the signs of
opioid exposure in themselves: light-headedness and euphoria.

If you work in emergency services, you
are likely working with a partner. Make sure
you and your partner have the same under-
standing of the risks at the scene, including
exposure to opioids.

**If you do not work in emergency ser-
vices,** you may be on your own. Consider
asking bystanders if they have training in
naloxone administration and could help you,
if needed. Narcan nasal spray makes it easy for
bystanders to help you. Equip bystanders who
offer to help with personal protective equipment (PPE), including those who offer CPR
assistance.

Cover your exposed skin and put on
personal protective equipment (PPE)

Any powder at a scene indicates a risk of
exposure and overdose to you, the rescuer.
Even small amounts of fentanyl, and minute
amounts of carfentanil, which are powerful

opioids common in the current opioid crisis, pose risks.

Even though you may not see powder at a scene, it's best to be cautious.

1. **Cover exposed skin** as best you can. Roll down your sleeves and button up your collar.

2. **Put on your PPE.** At minimum, this includes 2 pairs of nitrile gloves, safety-type glasses, and an N95 particulate respirator. If your job provides you with specialized respiration equipment, use it.

3. **Equip all assistants with PPE.** Anyone who assists you at the scene (e.g., a bystander who knows CPR) should cover their exposed skin and wear full PPE.

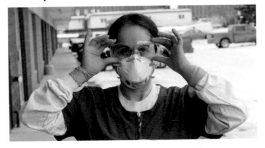

Full PPE: Everyone assisting at an opioid emergency scene should wear full PPE, including safety glasses, an N95 particulate respirator (at minimum), and 2 pairs of nitrile gloves. They should also cover as much exposed skin as possible.

COVID-19 and PPE

In treating people with possible COVID-19, public health agencies identify procedures that generate droplets as a particular risk to those providing care.[1,2] Cardiopulmonary resuscitation is considered a

procedure that generates droplets
[1,3] and it is often an essential procedure in responding to opioid emergencies.

The PPE that protects rescuers from accidental exposure to opioids also protects them from droplets, **except** that current guidelines also recommend gowns. The complete list of minimum recommended PPE is:[1,2]

- nitrile gloves (opioid emergencies require double gloving, which is more protection than required for droplet protection)
- safety glasses or eye shield (prescription eye glasses are not considered adequate protection)
- fit-tested N95 particulate respirator, or higher-level respirator
- gown

Stay up to date. Check online for updates from public health agencies in your jurisdiction for the latest recommendations on PPE during the pandemic. Also keep up to date on routine vaccines and specialized vaccines that may arise as this, and other viruses or bacteria, emerge and evolve.

Remove potential weapons on or near the person in crisis

Examples of potential weapons include heavy objects (e.g., tools), guns, knives, and needles. On regaining consciousness, a person in crisis may mistake help from a rescuer as aggression, or they may become aggressive because of opioid withdrawal or other drugs they have taken.

Consider soaking in water any visible powder

Powders on or near the person in crisis may contain opioids that you could accidently inhale. They pose less risk if they are wet.

If you do not work in emergency services, consider whether to withdraw to a safer location and call EMS (911). On-scene powder might make this the most sensible option.

Assist the person in crisis

1. **Assess level of consciousness.**
   - **Shout at the person.** Try to rouse them with verbal stimulus.
   - **Apply a painful stimulus.** If shouting doesn't work, pinch the tissues around the shoulders, or the back of the arms at the triceps (continue to shout). Pinch hard. Another method of painful stimulus is the sternal rub: using your knuckles, rub up and down on the person's breastbone while applying pressure.

2. **If the person is unresponsive, open the airway.**
   - Gently tilt the head back and lift up on the lower jaw (mandible). Tilting the head aligns the airway, and lifting the mandible lifts the tongue from the back of the airway (pharynx). The tongue is the number-one cause of airway obstruction in people who are unresponsive to verbal and painful stimulus.
   - *Do not take this step* if you suspect that the person has a spinal cord injury: use the modified jaw-thrust maneuver.

3. **Clear the mouth of obstructions.** This might include food, vomitus, or excess saliva. Removing obstructions may trigger a biting response, so stay alert and mind your fingers. To reduce the risk of a bite, gently open the lips and sweep your fingers on the inside of the cheeks, along the line where the cheek meets the jawbone (mandible).

   Note that, in some cases, once you've opened and cleared the airway, the person will begin to breathe on their own.

4. **Assess breathing and pulse.**
   - **If the person is breathing,** you need to assess if it is rapid enough and deep enough to sustain them. The average rate of breathing in adults is 12 to 20 ventilations per minute.

     › If you cannot remember the appropriate rate of breathing, consider this. If the person is breathing at an adequate rate and depth to keep them alive, their skin will be pink around the lips. If they are pale, this indicates shock. If they are pale and have blue coloring around the lips, they need assistance breathing.

   - **To check the pulse,** place your fingers on the carotid artery in the neck, next to the voice box (larynx). Take 5 to 10 seconds to feel for a pulse. If you feel a pulse, what is the rate? Is it fast or slow? A normal pulse in an adult is 60 to 100 beats per minute. Is the pulse strong or weak?

5. **If there is no pulse, begin CPR immediately at a rate of 30 chest compressions per 2 ventilations (30:2).**
   - **For chest compressions,** the target rate is 100 to 120 compressions per minute. Chest compressions circulate blood within the torso and the brain.
   - **For ventilations,** use a bag valve mask if this is an option for you (you need training in bag valve masks to use them properly). A bag valve mask lets you keep all your PPE on while assisting the person in crisis. Otherwise, use a barrier device (preferably a pocket mask with 1-way valve and mucus filter).

6. **If there is a pulse, but breathing is absent or inadequate, start rescue ventilations at a rate of 1 ventilation every 5 to 6 seconds.**

COVID-19, CPR, and ventilation assistance

If you work in emergency services, note that the Centers for Disease Control and Prevention recommend high-efficiency particulate air (HEPA) filters for expired air from bag valve masks.[1]

If you are any other kind of rescuer, consider providing hands-only CPR during the pandemic, as recommended by some agencies.[4]

- **This recommendation means you should not provide ventilation assistance via any kind of pocket mask** unless the COVID-19 status of the person in crisis is known to you. For example, the person in crisis may be a family member whom you know is negative for the virus.
- **In addition, consider placing a surgical mask (also known as a procedure mask) on the person in crisis before providing hands-only CPR.** This is because CPR is considered

a procedure that generates droplets,[1,3] which can contaminate rescuers, bystanders, and surfaces with the novel coronavirus. The mask should cover the nose and mouth of the person in crisis, so that it captures droplets that escape the person during chest compressions.

Stay up to date. Check online for updates from public health agencies in your jurisdiction for the latest recommendations on providing ventilation assistance during the pandemic.

7. **Administer naloxone.** A person in opioid crisis needs naloxone as soon as possible. Remember we discussed providing steps of care simultaneously? If you have bystanders on scene assisting with airway positioning or CPR, you can proceed more quickly to the administration of naloxone.

8. **Administer more naloxone as needed.** If in 3 to 5 minutes you do not observe an improvement in the person's condition, repeat the naloxone dose. If you are using an intranasal injection system (e.g., Narcan nasal spray), discharge the repeat dose in the opposite nostril.

   Overdoses with fentanyl, carfentanil, and other strong synthetic opioids may require 8 mg to 16 mg of naloxone to reverse (sometimes even higher doses). In terms of Narcan nasal spray, where each dispenser delivers a 4-mg dose, this is between 2 and 4 dispensers.

9. **Rule out other reasons for continued unconsciousness and respond appropriately.** If the person in crisis remains unconscious:
   • Check for injuries, such as head injuries and bleeding wounds.

- Check for a transdermal patch, including a fentanyl patch (prescribed for pain control) or a buprenorphine patch (prescribed for opioid addiction). Transdermal patches are applied to the skin to allow slow absorption of medication. Remove any fentanyl or buprenorphine patch that you find. Common locations for transdermal patches are the upper arm, chest, and back.
- Get information from bystanders about how the crisis happened.

10. **Watch for symptoms of mixed overdose.** If the person in crisis has taken other drugs in addition to opioids (resulting in a mixed overdose), the symptoms of the other drugs may emerge when you give naloxone. Note these symptoms: they provide clues about the situation of the person in crisis and the treatment they may ultimately need. They may also pose new crises for you to manage or threats to your safety.

    In some cases, hyperthermia (raised body temperature) may emerge. This requires first aid: place the person in crisis in the recovery position (provided they are breathing adequately) and pour water on the chest and back. Provide cool cloths.

    Sometimes, the new symptoms are hallucinations, delusions, or aggression. Do not attempt to restrain a person who becomes aggressive unless you are trained in restraint protocols. Talk to the person in a nonjudgmental manner and with calm reassurance. This can go a long way toward defusing aggression at an emergency scene until help arrives.

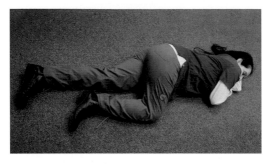

The recovery position: This position keeps the airway open and free of vomitus in an unconscious person.

Seek help if your health is at risk

If you have come in direct contact with an unknown powder at a scene, seek immediate help from EMS on scene, especially from dangerous goods personnel who may be responding from fire rescue. Risks from fentanyl and carfentanil powder can be reduced or eliminated with copious amounts of water. Soaking and rinsing exposed skin, eyes, and mucous membranes for several minutes may be significant in certain circumstances.

If you have a needlestick injury, seek immediate help.

- **If you work in EMS,** follow all protocols for needlestick injuries promptly.

- **If you are any other kind of rescuer:**
  › Seek immediate help from EMS if the injury may involve needles contaminated with synthetic opioids.
  › Seek help from a physician at an emergency department or clinic for any other kind of needlestick injury.

A note about needlestick injuries

Needlestick injuries come from accidental pokes with contaminated needles, which can infect you with HIV, hepatitis, and other infectious agents. Contaminated needles may be present at opioid emergency scenes because of drug paraphernalia, or because your naloxone kit is needle based.

Protocols for blood and body fluid exposure (BBFE), including needlestick injuries, have been in place for many years in health-care facilities. In other areas of work, protocols may or may not be in place. For example, they may not be in place in your job as a police, corrections, or security officer, or as a community outreach worker—even though you may, in these jobs, routinely respond to opioid emergencies in your community.

If your job routinely involves responding to opioid emergency scenes, check whether your job has a protocol in place for needlestick injuries. If not, work to get a protocol in place.

In the event of a needlestick injury, the immediate steps to reduce infection include:

- allowing the wound site to bleed
- using alcohol-based sanitizer on the wound site, until soap and water is available (note that alcohol-based hand sanitizer is not recommended for general decontamination at opioid emergency scenes)
- washing with soap and water as soon as possible

Depending on the situation, next steps may include drug prophylaxis in the form of retroviral medications to reduce the risk of hepatitis or HIV infection, and counseling.

The importance of needlestick-injury protocols cannot be overemphasized. If you receive a significant needlestick injury, and don't have a protocol in place, you may face delays in assessment and treatment of your injury. You will probably go a hospital emergency department, where you will complete sign-in procedures, undergo basic triage at the desk, and wait for a physician. Retroviral medications are critically important in cases of significant exposure, and should be started as soon as possible.

A protocol removes delays and barriers. Steps are spelled out, and everyone can immediately follow them to the letter. Care, lab work, counseling, and follow-up take place quickly and seamlessly, which reduces risk and stress in a stressful situation.

Dispose of hazardous materials

All used PPE and naloxone-delivery items are potentially infectious or a chemical risk. Discard and replace all items used to respond to an opioid emergency.

If you work in emergency services, follow protocols for disposing of dangerous goods, biohazards, and sharps.

If you are any other kind of rescuer, you will likely call EMS (911) for assistance. EMS, including ambulances and fire-rescue vehicles, have sharps containers for needles, and appropriate containers for contaminated clothing, equipment, and biohazards.

Decontaminate

1. **Remove contaminated clothing.** You may have been exposed to chemicals on scene, potentially fentanyl or carfentanil powder. Do not risk contaminating your home or workplace with clothing from the scene.

    If you work in emergency services, follow protocols in place for disposing of items contaminated with synthetic opioids.

    If you are any other kind of rescuer, seek help from EMS.

2. **Avoid alcohol-based hand sanitizers.** If you have particles of synthetic opioids (e.g., fentanyl or carfentanil) on your skin, alcohol-based sanitizers accelerate their absorption. You should also avoid hypochlorite bleach solutions for the same reason.

3. **Wash with soap and water as soon as possible.** Pay special attention to exposed skin.

COVID-19 and decontamination

Wash your hands with soap and water as soon as possible.

Avoid touching your face until you have washed your hands with soap and water. **This means: keep your eye protection and respirator on until you have washed your hands.**

Know and follow proper procedures for removing respirators. Check online for directions provided by the manufacturer.

After removing your PPE, wash your hands again.

Seek mental-health support as needed

Responding to overdoses in the community can be mentally distressing and traumatic. You are at particular risk of mental-health challenges, such as posttraumatic stress disorder, if your job routinely involves responding to opioid emergency scenes (e.g., health-care providers in emergency services; police, security, and corrections officers; community outreach workers). The current opioid crisis has increased the frequency of opioid emergencies in the community, and is taking a significant toll on the mental health of rescuers.

Stay alert to your mental health, including signs of mental-health challenges (e.g., trouble sleeping; substance dependency; unusual and persistent irritability or anxiety). Always reach out for help and support when you face challenges.

If you respond to opioid emergency scenes as part of a team, monitor your team members for signs of mental-health challenges. It is paramount for you and your team members to work closely together, and with mental-health services, to safeguard your mental health.

Responding to an opioid emergency scene in the community: law-enforcement, security, and corrections officers

If you work in law enforcement, security, or corrections, you are often the first rescuers on the scene of emergencies that involve opioids. This puts you at higher risk of accidental opioid exposure.

You can use your special training in scene assessment, situational awareness, self-protection, and self-directed first aid when responding to opioid emergencies.

Phases of an emergency

As a military tactical problem, an opioid emergency has 3 distinct phases.

1. **Active phase:** The scene is not safe or contained. Risks from persons, the scene, weapons, glass, needles, and so on are not yet controlled. Frontline responders work

to secure the scene, make it safe, remove threats, and provide first aid to those in need.

2. **Tactical phase:** Initial threats have been controlled. Everyone is wearing PPE, all persons who posed a risk have been dealt with, and the team can continue care of those in need. This phase can change at any time, so frontline responders need to remain alert, maintain heightened situational awareness, and provide oversight and support for team members directly involved in the care of person(s) in crisis. If all goes well, this phase evolves into the evacuation phase.

3. **Evacuation phase:** EMS and firefighters are involved in secondary assessment and care of person(s) in crisis. Frontline responders have made the scene safe, accounted for threats, and now assist in the handoff of those requiring medical care and transport to hospital.

Self-care and buddy care

Here's a situation you might encounter as a police officer. You and your partner are conducting the arrest of an impaired driver. As you pull the suspect from the car, a large bag of powder breaks and the powder becomes airborne. You inhale some of the powder. You and your partner are still working to secure the suspect when you realize that you feel light-headed and euphoric. You call out to alert your partner of your situation.

Self-care and *buddy care* are military terms that describe how and when to apply first aid.

Self-care describes the life-saving interventions you, as a rescuer, may need to provide to yourself. In tactical and challenging environments, you may be alone, or your team members may be too busy with other threats to provide care if you go down.

Your personal first-aid kit (PFAK) is key. This is likely a kit that you assemble for yourself, and that each of your team members assembles for themselves. Each PFAK should contain 2 to 4 Narcan nasal spray dispensers, among other equipment. These are *for your use first*. They are often used on members of the public, but their purpose is, first, self-care, and second, care of a team member (buddy care).

Steps for self-care administration of Narcan nasal spray

1. **Recognize the threat.** Stay alert to signs of opioid exposure: light-headedness and euphoria.

2. **Alert your team members of your situation.** Ensure EMS (911) has been called.

3. **Withdraw to fresh air.** Take this step only if you can remain safe.

4. **Access your Narcan nasal spray**.

5. **Kneel or lie down.** You do not want to lose consciousness from a standing position, but take this step only if you can remain safe.

6. **Administer Narcan nasal spray up a nostril, and press the nostril closed.** If you can, lie in the recovery position to ensure your airway is open if you lose consciousness.

7. **Administer more Narcan nasal spray as needed.** If you are not feeling better in 2 to 5 minutes, give yourself another dose in the opposite nostril.

8. **Remove your body armor.** Take this step only if you can remain safe. Removing body armor will allow you to breathe easier. Remember that opioids affect your ability to breathe. Tight-fitting uniforms and body armor are not helpful in this situation.

   If it is not safe to remove your body armor, loosen the Velcro straps that hold it tight to your body. This leaves the panels in place for safety, but allows your chest wall to move freely.

Steps for buddy care

When it is safe to approach your team member, you can provide buddy care. Ensure that you are not exposed to on-scene threats, and that you are wearing PPE as necessary. Make sure you have your own PFAK available.

Use the PFAK of your team member to help your team member, *not your own PFAK*. Only when the PFAK of your team member is exhausted should you use your own PFAK. This may seem selfish or uncaring, but you must be able to function and care for yourself, or you will not be able to support the operation.

1. **Ensure that assistance is on the way.** Make sure appropriate resources are en route, such as EMS and a dangerous goods team. Note that dangerous goods teams respond to emergencies where large amounts of opioids are present (e.g., drug manufacturing labs).

2. **Put on your PPE.**

3. **Approach your team member.** Assure them that the scene is now safe and you are there to provide care.

4. **If you suspect the scene is contaminated, drag your team member away from the threat.** Try to choose a location, such as a corner, that provides you with a good view of the overall scene.

5. **Consider disarming your team member.** Examples of weapons include sidearms, knifes, and batons. Exposure to airborne drugs could involve opioids, methamphetamine, or cocaine: any of these drugs, alone or in combination, could render your team member incapable of distinguishing a friendly approach from a threatening one.

6. **Work from the apex of your team member.** Take this step only if you can remain safe. In the apex position, you kneel behind the head. This allows you to look down the body, maintain situational awareness of the scene, and protect the head and neck of your team member.

7. **Consider soaking with water any visible powder on your team member.** This reduces your risk of exposure to opioids and other drugs.

8. **Check your team member's level of consciousness (LOC) and check their airway, breathing, and circulation (ABCs).** If needed, access the body armor, remove the Velcro holding the armor in place, and flip the chest panel back. This allows you to kneel on a safe surface, protected from needles, glass, and other potential hazards. This

also allows your team member to breathe easier.

9. **Access your team member's PFAK.** Use theirs first, not yours.

10. **Provide support as needed.** Support could include doses of naloxone, or ventilation assistance with a bag valve mask. If CPR chest compressions are needed, and you are alone, they can be done from the apex position until help arrives. The apex position allows you to maintain situational awareness, without placing your back to possible threats, as the scene evolves.

K-9 opioid emergencies

Tactical teams often have dogs as members. In many law-enforcement and security applications, dogs do their primary work with their noses. Contact with, and inhalation of, fentanyl or carfentanil powders or liquids could be life-threatening.

Prepare for the possibility of exposure. It is important to have a procedure in place with the veterinarian attached to your agency. K-9 team members should also have their own PFAK, which their handlers should carry.

Dogs in opioid crisis need care and intervention the same as humans. If a K-9 team member loses consciousness, has slowed breathing, and shows signs and symptoms of overdose like a human, give them naloxone. In most cases, using Narcan nasal spray can be safe and effective for dogs. Follow up with the veterinarian as soon as possible.

Decontamination of the dog must also occur. Flushing with water at the scene of an emergency renders most opioid powders and liquids inert. Most veterinarians recommend a follow-up shower with soap and water to remove all traces from fur and skin.

11. **Continue care until help arrives.** Ensure all emergency services personnel are warned of threats on scene before they arrive.

12. **Reassess and monitor your team member.** Take this step only if you can remain safe. Complete a thorough head-to-toe physical examination to rule out injuries such as cuts or fractures. Cover your team member with a thermal barrier to preserve and contain precious body heat.

Responding to an emergency scene in the community: health-care providers in emergency services

The situations you encounter as a health-care provider in emergency services may involve scenes where rescuers are already in place and helping a person in crisis. Or you may be called to a scene by someone who feels a situation is too dangerous for them to intervene.

The general procedures for responding to opioid emergency scenes apply to you: scene assessment; coordination with your team members; full PPE; CPR and repeated naloxone administration, as needed, for the person(s) in crisis; disposal of hazardous materials; and decontamination.

In addition, if other rescuers are in place, you need to attend to them as well as the person(s) in crisis. This is because rescuers on scene may have been exposed to opioids, or they may have needlestick injuries. They may need help with decontamination, and they will need help disposing of used rapid response equipment.

Continue to wear your full PPE until your risk of exposure to opioids from the scene, person(s) in crisis, and on-scene rescuers is over.

To assist rescuers on scene:

1. **Ask about possible opioid exposure.** Respond as necessary. Check rescuers for symptoms of opioid exposure.

2. **Ask about needlestick injuries.** Any rescuer with a significant needlestick injury needs immediate care from a physician.

3. **Assist with decontamination.** For example, advise any rescuer exposed to powdered forms of opioids to remove contaminated clothing. Help them bag or box the clothing, or direct them to an on-scene dangerous goods team. Follow the protocols in your jurisdiction for disposing of items contaminated with synthetic opioids.

4. **Locate and dispose of used PPE and naloxone-delivery items.** Follow the protocols in your jurisdiction for disposing of items contaminated with synthetic opioids.

Responding to arrivals from an opioid emergency scene in the community

From an emergency scene, a person in crisis may arrive at a hospital ER, or a community medical clinic or outreach center. They may arrive by ambulance, or friends and family may bring them.

A person who arrives from the scene of an opioid emergency is not properly decontaminated. They may have fentanyl or carfentanil powder on their clothing, or in their hair or pockets. They may also be carrying their own contaminated shooting kits with needles and syringes, or other drugs.

If you are a health-care provider in an ER, make sure you have easy access to a regularly maintained naloxone kit and PPE. It is paramount to heighten your awareness of risk and use all PPE as provided. All team members in the room should wear appropriate PPE. This includes:

- 2 pairs of properly fitting nitrile gloves (double glove)
- a disposable gown with long sleeves (at minimum, roll down the sleeves you have on and do up your collar)
- an N95 particulate respirator with eye shield, or safety glasses with a regular N95 particulate respirator (all types of respirators require fit testing)

If you are a health-care provider in a community medical clinic, such as a doctor's office or walk-in clinic, make sure your workplace has well-placed, well-marked, and regularly maintained rapid response equipment, including full PPE and a naloxone kit. Every community medical clinic and walk-in clinic ought to have rapid response equipment, but many do not.

- Practice using the naloxone-delivery system in your kit by using sample delivery systems.
- Heighten your awareness of risk from opioid crises, and use caution and full PPE if you think you are dealing with an opioid crisis.
- Ensure everyone who helps you assist a person in crisis wears full PPE.

If you are a community outreach worker, you may have rapid response equipment in place. Check to make sure. In addition:

- Practice using the naloxone-delivery system in your kit by using sample delivery systems.
- Heighten your awareness of risk from opioid crises, and use caution and full PPE if you think you are dealing with an opioid crisis.
- Ensure everyone who helps you assist a person in crisis wears full PPE.

COVID-19 and arrivals from emergency scenes

The COVID-19 status of a person who arrives at your ER, medical clinic, or outreach center may not be known. Stay up to date with, and follow, the public health guidelines in your jurisdiction that apply to your facility or workplace. As with all situations in health care, assuming all patients are potentially infectious is a standard approach. COVID-19 and influenza patients have heightened the awareness of, and need for, appropriate PPE, training, and drills.

Pediatric opioid emergencies

The steps for assisting a child or infant in opioid overdose are similar to the steps for assisting an adult.

A key similarity is naloxone dose. Naloxone doses are the same for infants and children as for adults.[5] Infants and children do not require smaller doses. They do, however, require shorter needles for intramuscular (IM) injection, because infants and children have less muscle tissue than adults. If you anticipate rescuing children in crisis and you work with IM-administered naloxone, include 1-inch (2.5-cm) needles in your rapid response equipment.

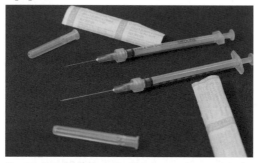

Comparing needle lengths: This image shows a 1-inch (2.5-cm) needle and a 1.5-inch (40-mm) needle. Use the shorter needle for children. (The shorter needle is also suitable for adults with less muscle or fat tissue.)

A key difference is CPR technique and equipment. CPR for pediatric and infant patients requires specific training. Most CPR courses include pediatric CPR, but may not include infant CPR. For the purposes of CPR:

- an infant is younger than 1 year of age

- a child is 1 year of age to when signs of puberty are apparent

In addition, you need pediatric bag valve masks if you anticipate rescuing children in opioid crisis. These are smaller than adult-size bag valve masks: they fit the smaller size of children's faces, and they deliver a smaller ventilation per squeeze.

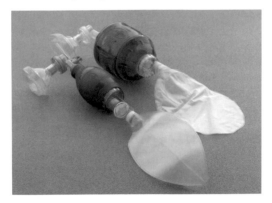

Pediatric bag valve mask: The bag valve mask on the left is for pediatric use. Children need smaller bag valve masks than adults.

Pediatric rapid response sequence

Here's the entire sequence for responding to an opioid emergency where the person in crisis is a child or infant.

Assess the scene.

Call EMS (911).

Work with a buddy if possible.

Cover your exposed skin and put on PPE.

Remove potential weapons on or near the child in crisis.

Consider soaking in water any visible powder.

Assist the child in crisis.

1. Assess level of consciousness.
   - Shout at the child.
   - Apply a painful stimulus.

2. If the child is unresponsive, open the airway.

3. Clear the mouth of obstructions.

4. Assess breathing and pulse.

   Children and infants have higher respiration rates than adults. Keep this in mind when assessing their breathing. Check for signs of inadequate respiration: pale skin and blue coloring around the lips.

   Children and infants have higher pulse rates than adults:

   - children: 80 to 140 beats per minute (the older the child, the lower the rate)
   - infants: 100 to 180 beats per minute (the older the infant, the lower the rate)

   Note that pulse assessment in infants requires assessing the brachial pulse on the

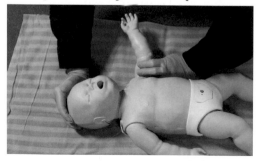

Brachial pulse check in an infant: Place 2 fingers on the inner upper arm.

inner upper arm. Infants have short necks and fatty neck tissue, which make carotid pulse checks difficult.

5. **If there is no pulse, begin CPR immediately.**
   - With 1 rescuer, the rate is 30 chest compressions per 2 ventilations (30:2).
   - With 2 rescuers, the rate is 15 chest compressions per 2 ventilations (15:2).

   Use a pediatric bag valve mask if you have one and are trained to use it.

6. **If there is a pulse, but breathing is absent or inadequate, start rescue ventilations.**
   Children and infants require more frequent ventilations than adults:
   - children: 16 to 24 ventilations per minute
   - infants: 24+ ventilations per minute

7. **Administer naloxone.**
   Give infants and children the same dose you would give an adult. For IM injection, use a 1-inch (2.5-cm) needle.

8. **Administer more naloxone as needed.**
   Give infants and children the same repeat doses you would give an adult.

9. **Rule out other reasons for continued unconsciousness and respond appropriately.**

10. **Watch for symptoms of mixed overdose.**

Seek help if your health is at risk.
Dispose of hazardous materials.
Decontaminate.
Seek mental-health support as needed.

REFERENCES

1 Centers for Disease Control and Prevention. Interim guidance for
   emergency medical services (EMS) and 911 public safety answering
   points (PSAPS) for COVID-19 in the United States [Internet]. [Atlanta
   (GA)]: CDC; [updated 2020 10 March; cited 2020 15 April]. Available
   from https://www.cdc.gov/coronavirus/2019-ncov/hcp/guidance-for-
   ems.html

2 Public Health Agency of Canada. Corona virus (COVID-19): For health
   professionals [Internet]. [Ottawa (ON)]: The Agency; [updated 2020
   April 11; cited 2020 April 15]. Available from https://www.canada.ca/
   en/public-health/services/diseases/2019-novel-coronavirus-infection/
   health-professionals.html?topic=tilelink

3 Public Health Ontario. IPAC recommendations for use of personal
   protective equipment for care of individuals with suspect or confirmed
   COVID-19 [Internet]. [Toronto (ON)]: Public Health Ontario; [updated
   2020 April 6; cited 2020 April 15]. Available from https://www.
   publichealthontario.ca/-/media/documents/ncov/updated-ipac-
   measures-covid-19.pdf?la=en

4 Heart and Stroke Foundation of Canada. Modifications to public
   hands-only CPR during the COVID-19 pandemic [Internet].
   Ottawa (ON): The Foundation; [updated 2020 6 April; cited 2020
   April 15]. Available from https://www.heartandstroke.ca/articles/
   modification-to-hands-only-cpr-during-the-covid-19-pandemic

5 Boyer EW. Management of opioid analgesic overdose. N Engl J Med.
   2012 July;367(2):146–155.

4

Complications in opioid emergencies

This chapter covers some complications you might encounter when assisting a person in crisis at an opioid emergency scene in the community.

The person doesn't respond to naloxone

There are several reasons a person in crisis might not respond to naloxone.

- **The overdose involves powerful synthetic opioids.** Opioid overdoses involving synthetic opioids, such as fentanyl and carfentanil, sometimes require more than 16 mg of naloxone to reverse.

- **It's a mixed overdose.** In addition to opioids, the person may have taken other drugs that depress the central nervous system (CNS). Naloxone neutralizes the effect of opioids (temporarily), but not nonopioid CNS depressants (e.g., alcohol, benzodiazepines). Note, however, that naloxone remains crucial first aid in this situation. See Chapter 5 for more information.

- **It's not an opioid crisis.** A person might exhibit symptoms that resemble opioid overdose because of conditions such as:
  › diabetic emergency, including hypoglycemia and hyperglycemia
  › stroke
  › infections of the brain, such as encephalitis and meningitis
  › brain injury
  › exposure to toxins or poisons
  › hypothermia or hyperthermia
  › hypoxia (low levels of oxygen in the blood)
  › epilepsy
  › dementia-related disorders
  › cardiac emergencies, such as heart attack

- **The person has nasal structural abnormalities.** This is an issue for rescuers administering naloxone by nasal spray. This is why you use the opposite nostril when you give a person in crisis a repeat dose of naloxone.

What to do

- **Give repeat doses of naloxone.** Some overdoses involving synthetic opioids require a total of 8 mg to 16 mg of naloxone (and occasionally more) to reverse. Provide naloxone even if you are not sure why a person is in crisis: naloxone has minimally significant side effects if given when not required. Follow this rule of thumb: when in doubt, give naloxone

- **If you are administering naloxone by nasal spray, switch nostrils for repeat doses.**

- **Rule out other causes of continued unconsciousness.**
  - › Check for injuries, such as head injuries and bleeding wounds.
  - › Check for a transdermal patch, including a fentanyl patch (prescribed for pain control) or a buprenorphine patch (prescribed for opioid addiction). Transdermal patches are applied to the skin to allow slow absorption of medication. Remove any fentanyl or buprenorphine patch that you find. Common locations for transdermal patches are the upper arm, chest, and back.
  - › Get information from bystanders about how the crisis happened.

The person has vomited

Vomiting is common in opioid overdoses: opioids suppress the gag reflex, which means a person in crisis often regurgitates their stomach contents. Stay alert to signs that the person in crisis has vomited even if you don't see vomitus: listen for gurgling sounds.

What to do

- **Clear the mouth and airway** of a person in crisis so they don't inhale vomitus or other materials. Inhaled material can lead to lung infections, such as aspiration pneumonia.
- **Mind your fingers.** Clearing the mouth and airway can trigger a bite reflex.

The person becomes hyperthermic after naloxone

Hyperthermia is elevated body temperature. It can lead to seizures, brain damage, and death.

In opioid crises, hyperthermia can occur in mixed overdoses involving CNS stimulants such as gamma-hydroxybutyrate (GHB), MDMA (3,4-methylenedioxymethamphetamine or ecstasy), and cocaine.

It can also happen if opioids are combined with antidepressants such as selective serotonin reuptake inhibitors (SSRIs).

What to do

- Cooling a hyperthermic patient is critically important. Place the person in crisis in the recovery position (provided they are breathing adequately) and pour water on the chest and back. Provide cool cloths.

The person becomes combative after naloxone

This can happen in some mixed overdoses involving opioids and drugs with behavioral effects, such as GHB or methamphetamine.

It can also happen when naloxone triggers withdrawal symptoms in opioid addicts.

What to do

- **Before you assist any person in crisis, remove potential weapons on or near the person.** This includes heavy objects (e.g., tools), guns, knives, and needles.
- **Do not attempt to restrain a person in crisis unless you are trained in restraint protocols.** Talk to the person in a nonjudgmental manner and with calm reassurance. This can go a long way toward defusing aggression at an emergency scene until help arrives.

The person in opioid crisis is also injured

A person in crisis may fall when they lose consciousness and injure themselves. Or they may have a bleeding wound from an altercation that took place before they lost consciousness.

What to do

- Ideally, several rescuers could respond to this situation at once (e.g., to administer naloxone, provide ventilations, and stop bleeding).
- If you are the only rescuer, provide naloxone first and then follow your cardiopulmonary resuscitation (CPR) training to provide first aid until help arrives.

5

Mixed overdoses: opioids with other drugs

A mixed overdose scenario

Consider this scenario: you are on the scene of a person found unconscious and unresponsive. You have assessed the scene for safety, called emergency medical services (EMS: 911), and put on full personal protective equipment (PPE). You approach the person and assess their level of consciousness, and their airway, breathing, and pulse. They are unconscious and completely unresponsive to verbal and physical stimulation. Their airway is partially obstructed with saliva, which you clear (being careful to avoid triggering a bite response). Their breathing is slow and very shallow. Their pulse is slow and weak.

These symptoms are consistent with opioid overdose. Opioids are central nervous system (CNS) depressants: they reduce level of consciousness, threaten the airway, and decrease breathing and pulse rates.

You administer Narcan nasal spray. You decide that the rate and depth of ventilations is not enough to sustain life. You assist ventilations with a bag valve mask. After 3 to 5 minutes of assisted ventilations, you note a slight improvement in their breathing rate and depth. However, they are not moving, and have not regained consciousness. You administer a second dose of Narcan nasal spray in the opposite nostril. After several more minutes, the rate and depth of ventilations improve. The person is now breathing on their own at 12 breaths per minute and maintaining pink skin.

You place the person in the recovery position and await EMS. Despite improvement in vital signs, you note that the person remains heavily sedated, though more responsive than at first. When you apply painful stimulus with a triceps pinch, they now react to the pain. They are still sedated but responsive to pain when EMS arrives.

This scenario is an example of a mixed, or polypharmacy, overdose involving opioids, where a person in crisis has taken opioids together with other drugs. Mixed overdoses are common in the current opioid crisis. In some cases, people don't realize that recreational and illicit drugs, such as benzodiazepines, cannabis, and cocaine, are often mixed with powerful synthetic opioids. In other cases, people may choose to take these drugs despite knowing they are laced. In addition, some people deliberately take opioids on top of other drugs, such as alcohol or antidepressants, because they don't realize the risk or because they choose to ignore the risk.

How naloxone affects mixed overdoses

Any apparent opioid overdose at an emergency scene could be a mixed overdose. This possibility does not alter the way you respond. **Always administer naloxone when a person in crisis has symptoms consistent with opioid overdose.**

However, stay alert to how naloxone affects the person in crisis. In mixed overdoses, the drug of highest concentration usually dominates the symptoms you observe. So, in a mixed overdose where an opioid has the highest concentration, you will likely observe symptoms consistent with opioid overdose. When you administer naloxone in this situation, the naloxone neutralizes the opioid (at least temporarily) and the effects of the next symptom-dominating drug may emerge.

If the next symptom-dominating drug is a CNS depressant, naloxone will probably improve the person's symptoms, but not as much as you expect. The person, for example, may not regain consciousness, even on repeat naloxone. The scenario that starts this chapter is an example of this situation.

If the next symptom-dominating drug is a CNS stimulant, naloxone may reveal symptoms opposite to an opioid overdose: the person may become conscious and agitated, with rapid breathing and a rapid pulse.

If the next symptom-dominating drug alters perceptions or behavior, naloxone may reveal symptoms such as hallucinations, delusions, paranoia, or aggression.

First-aid alerts for responding to mixed overdoses

It is crucial to follow the procedures presented in this guide for responding to opioid emergency scenes. These procedures help you respond safely and effectively.

Before you assist a person in crisis, always: assess the scene for safety, call EMS (911), and put on full PPE. Work with a buddy, if possible, and make sure they wear full PPE, too. Remove any potential weapons on or near the person in crisis. See Chapter 3 of this guide for complete information.

When you assist a person in crisis, be aware that you may be dealing with a mixed overdose. You may not know this until after you administer naloxone.

Always administer naloxone for signs and symptoms consistent with opioid overdose.

Note changes in signs and symptoms that emerge after naloxone administration. These changes are clues about the situation of the person in crisis, and the treatment they may ultimately need. In addition, you may need to respond to emerging symptoms.

Get information from bystanders. Does anyone know what the person consumed? Did anyone see the person lose consciousness? If loss of consciousness was sudden and followed use of a possible opioid, consider opioid overdose likely. Information from bystanders can prepare you for the symptoms of the next symptom-dominating drug.

Rule out other causes of continued unconsciousness. If a person remains unconscious after naloxone administration:

- Check for injuries, such as head injuries and bleeding wounds.
- Check for a transdermal patch, including a fentanyl patch (prescribed for pain control) or a buprenorphine patch (prescribed for opioid addiction). Transdermal patches are applied to the skin to allow slow absorption of medication. Remove any fentanyl or buprenorphine patch that you find. Common locations for transdermal patches are the upper arm, chest, and back.

Pay particular attention to the airway in any person who remains unconscious. Closely monitor their airway, breathing, and circulation (ABCs). Even if they begin breathing on their own, ensure their ability to maintain an airway. Stay alert to regurgitation and vomiting, which is common in overdose situations: an unconscious person can aspirate vomitus into their lungs.

Drugs commonly mixed with opioids

Alcohol

What is alcohol?

Alcohol (ethanol) is a CNS depressant.

Alcohol and opioids are taken together quite often. People taking pain-control medications may drink alcohol, which can lead to mixed overdose. Because both substances are CNS depressants, the risk is significant. A person who consumes alcohol and takes a drug laced with synthetic opioids (e.g., fentanyl or carfentanil) is especially vulnerable to CNS depression.

Signs and symptoms of alcohol use

The signs and symptoms of alcohol consumption vary from person to person and with circumstances. Impairment depends on blood-alcohol concentration (BAC), which can be measured. BAC increases as alcohol is metabolized in the digestive system, which means the effects of alcohol can take time to manifest. A person already in crisis may become worse as they digest and absorb the alcohol they have recently consumed.

Alcohol taken alone would reveal the following signs and symptoms in the average person:

- elevated or depressed mood
- loss of coordination and motor control

- decreased consciousness, ranging from tired to unconscious
- reduced respiration, ranging from slowed breathing, to irregular breathing, to cessation of breathing (in severe cases)
- dehydration
- decreased body temperature, potentially leading to hypothermia
- cool, clammy, and possibly blue-colored (cyanotic) skin
- vomiting, leading to airway obstruction and risk of aspiration of stomach contents into the lungs

Benzodiazepines

What are benzodiazepines?
Benzodiazepines are CNS depressants.

In medicine, they are commonly used in an array of contexts, such as management of seizures, anxiety, panic attacks, alcohol withdrawal, insomnia, bipolar and personality disorders, depression, epilepsy, tinnitus (ringing in the ears), and movement disorders. They are also used for sedation prior to medical procedures.

As illicit drugs, they are pills, taken orally. "Benzos" are either stolen from the legal chain of supply or counterfeited outside the legal chain of supply. Counterfeits can be laced with synthetic opioids, such as fentanyl and carfentanil.

Signs and symptoms of benzodiazepine use

- decreased consciousness: drowsiness, slurred speech
- confusion
- dizziness
- trembling
- impaired coordination
- impaired vision

Buprenorphine

What is buprenorphine?
Buprenorphine is a CNS depressant.

In medicine, it is used to treat opioid addiction, and is often combined with naloxone in a single medication (buprenorphine-naloxone). It is a type of opioid, and is considered an improved and safer version of methadone (mixed overdoses with methadone also occur, but are less common). It is available on prescription for self-administration, and dispensed in community-treatment centers, detention centers, and prisons.

Buprenorphine comes as a pill and a transdermal patch. In health-care settings, it may be administered by injection. It has several trade names: Subutex and Buprenex are buprenorphine-only medications; Suboxone, Bunavail, and Zubsolv are buprenorphine-naloxone medications.

As an illicit drug, buprenorphine pills are generally sold or given away by people who have prescriptions. The pills may be crushed and snorted or smoked, or dissolved and injected. The risk of overdose from buprenorphine-only pills increases with crushed-pill methods of consumption. Addicts also sometimes combine buprenorphine with other opioids to increase their high.

Signs and symptoms of buprenorphine abuse

- decreased level of consciousness
- decreased respiration
- decreased heart rate and pulse strength
- irregular heartbeat (dysrhythmia)
- euphoria, calmness
- apparent intoxication (the person appears drunk)
- headache, dizziness, sleepiness, blurred vision
- pinpoint pupils
- nausea and vomiting
- mood swings

First-aid alerts for buprenorphine

People addicted to opioids are among those who abuse buprenorphine. When an opioid addict receives naloxone, they may go into opioid withdrawal.

In addition, if addicts crush and consume buprenorphine-naloxone pills (as opposed to buprenorphine-only pills), they may experience intense opioid-withdrawal symptoms.[1]

Symptoms of opioid withdrawal include:

- tremors (shaking)

- muscle twitching
- yawning
- watery eyes
- runny nose
- goose bumps
- increased heart rate, pulse strength, and blood pressure
- increased respiration rate
- abdominal cramps
- dilated pupils
- nausea and vomiting
- diarrhea
- anxiety

In some cases, addicts may become combative. Do not attempt to restrain a person in crisis unless you are trained in restraint protocols. Talk to the person in a nonjudgmental manner and with calm reassurance. This can go a long way toward defusing aggression at an emergency scene until help arrives.

Cannabis

What is cannabis?
Cannabis is a psychoactive drug.

It comes from the plant *Cannabis sativa*. Its main psychoactive component is tetrahydrocannabinol (THC). Hashish, or hash, has a higher concentration of THC than other forms of cannabis.

As a recreational or illicit drug, cannabis can be eaten or smoked (hashish is usually smoked). It goes by a variety of names, including weed, ganga, hash, Mary Jane, pot, reefer, hooch, toke, and others.

In certain forms, cannabis is legal in Canada and parts of the United States. As well, components of the cannabis plant are used in medications to treat pain, nausea and vomiting, loss of appetite, and glaucoma. Researchers are currently exploring other medical uses.

Illicit cannabis can be laced with synthetic opioids, such as fentanyl and carfentanil. Fentanyl and carfentanil mixed with cannabis has led to many overdoses and deaths.

Signs and symptoms of cannabis use
Taken on its own, cannabis can have the following effects:

- euphoria, calmness
- paranoia
- increased heart rate
- red eyes
- hunger
- muscle weakness
- tremors (shaking)

When taken with opioids, cannabis adds to the depressive effects of opioids on the central nervous system.

Cocaine and crack cocaine

What is cocaine?
Cocaine is a powerful CNS stimulant.

It comes from the coca plant. Indigenous Peoples in South and Central America have used coca for thousands of years in tea, or by consuming the leaves. Cocaine was first isolated from the leaves in 1860.[2]

In medicine, cocaine is used to control nasal bleeding and nasal pain, and as a numbing agent.

As an illicit drug, it can be a powder, which can be snorted, or a liquid, which can be injected. In "rock" form, it can be superheated and smoked as crack. It is often laced with synthetic opioids, such as fentanyl and carfentanil.

Signs and symptoms of cocaine use
- increased heart rate, pulse strength, and blood pressure
- increased body temperature (hyperthermia)
- increased respiration rate
- dilated pupils
- sweating
- euphoria
- agitation

First-aid alerts for cocaine
Cocaine use can cause a significant rise in body temperature (hyperthermia), which can lead to seizures, brain damage, and death if not corrected. Cooling a hyperthermic patient is critically important. Place the person in crisis in the recovery position (provided they are breathing adequately) and pour water on the chest and back. Provide cool cloths.

Cocaine use sometimes leads to heart attack or stroke.

Gamma-hydroxybutyrate (GHB)

What is GHB?

GHB is a CNS depressant.

GHB is a neurotransmitter that occurs naturally in the human body. It produces similar effects to opioids.

In medicine, it is used to treat narcolepsy (a sleeping disorder).

As an illicit drug, it is taken in liquid, powder, or pill form. It goes by many names: G, candy raver, cherry meth, grievous bodily harm, liquid E, liquid ecstasy, scoop, and more. It is popular as a club and rave drug. It is also a date-rape drug. Some bodybuilders use it illegally from an (unfounded) belief that it builds muscle, similar to steroids.

Signs and symptoms of GHB use

- euphoria
- decreased consciousness, coma, and seizures
- amnesia
- nausea and vomiting
- decreased body temperature (hypothermia)
- decreased respiration, leading to respiratory arrest
- decreased heart rate, pulse strength, and blood pressure
- irregular heartbeat (dysrhythmia)
- aggressive behaviors and possible hallucinations
- dilated pupils

First-aid alerts for GHB

Research has demonstrated that people who
are recovering from a GHB overdose may
wake up abruptly and exhibit aggression. In
health-care settings, they may remove their
own breathing tubes and aspirate stomach
contents into their lungs. When aggressive,
they can pose a risk to nearby caregivers.
Do not attempt to restrain a person in crisis
unless you are trained in restraint protocols.
Talk to the person in a nonjudgmental manner and with calm reassurance. This can go
a long way toward defusing aggression at an
emergency scene until help arrives.

Naloxone is beneficial in overdoses involving only GHB. Although GHB does not attach
to opioid receptors directly (unlike opioids),
it extends its effects by other mechanisms in
the body.

Ketamine

What is ketamine?

Ketamine is a CNS depressant.

In medicine, it is a veterinary anesthetic
and painkiller. Until recently, veterinary medicine was its primary use. It is now also exten-
sively used in human medicine by paramedics
and in hospitals.

As an illicit drug, it can be eaten, snorted,
or injected. It is goes by several names, including special K, vitamin K, K, jet, ket, green,
and cat valium. It has been used illegally since
the 1970s. The onset of effects ranges from

immediate to 30 minutes, depending on how it is taken. It is a date-rape drug. In addition to opioids, it may be mixed with MDMA (ecstasy), marijuana, alcohol, and lysergic acid diethylamide (LSD).

Signs and symptoms of ketamine use

- hallucinations
- delirium
- nausea and vomiting
- impaired respiration, from difficulty breathing to complete respiratory arrest
- a sense of being "near death" or "out of body" (users call this the "k-hole")
- muscle rigidity
- paranoia
- increased heart rate, pulse strength, and blood pressure
- loss of ability to move or speak

First-aid alerts for ketamine

Users often take high doses of ketamine to reach the "k-hole," which can lead to respiratory arrest and cardiac arrest. Combined with opioids, and possibly alcohol or other drugs, ketamine is truly a risk to life.

MDMA (ecstasy)

What is MDMA?

MDMA (3,4-methylenedioxymethamphetamine) is a CNS stimulant (it is an analogue of amphetamine).

In medicine, amphetamines are used in to treat conditions such as attention deficit hyperactivity disorder and narcolepsy.

As an illicit drug, MDMA is a pill or gel cap, or a powder that is snorted. Its names include dance drug, love drug, E, XTC, ex, and molly. It can be laced with synthetic opioids, such as fentanyl and carfentanil.

Signs and symptoms of MDMA use

- euphoria and reduced inhibition
- sexual arousal (possible)
- altered mental status: loss of sense of time
- involuntary clenching of the teeth
- dilated pupils
- muscle cramps

MDMA overdose causes a hypermetabolic state, which can emerge on administration of naloxone in a mixed overdose with the following signs and symptoms:

- increased body temperature (hyperthermia)
- dehydration
- seizures, leading to unconsciousness
- increased heart rate, pulse strength, and blood pressure
- irregular heartbeat (dysrhythmia)
- sweating
- diarrhea
- involuntary movements

First-aid alerts for MDMA

MDMA overdose can cause a significant rise in body temperature (hyperthermia), which can lead to seizures, brain damage, and death if not corrected. Cooling a hyperthermic patient is critically important. Place the person in crisis in the recovery position (provided they are breathing adequately) and pour water on the chest and back. Provide cool cloths.

Methamphetamine

What is methamphetamine?

Methamphetamine is a powerful CNS stimulant (it is an analogue of amphetamine).

In medicine, amphetamines are used in to treat conditions such as attention deficit hyperactivity disorder and narcolepsy. Methamphetamine was also used to keep soldiers awake and alert during World War II.

As an illicit drug, it is a pill taken orally; or a powder that is snorted or smoked, or dissolved in a liquid and injected; or a crystal (crystal meth) that is smoked. It has several names including meth, crystal meth, and others.

Signs and symptoms of methamphetamine use

- increased heart rate, pulse strength, and blood pressure
- increased body temperature (hyperthermia)
- increased respiration rate

- paranoia and delusions
- hallucinations
- violent behavior
- euphoria
- increased alertness
- sweating
- impaired coordination
- twitching and picking at skin
- dilated pupils

First-aid alerts for methamphetamine

Methamphetamine overdose can cause a significant rise in body temperature (hyperthermia), which can lead to seizures, brain damage, and death if not corrected. Cooling a hyperthermic patient is critically important. Place the person in crisis in the recovery position (provided they are breathing adequately) and pour water on the chest and back. Provide cool cloths.

Meth users may become combative. Do not attempt to restrain a person in crisis unless you are trained in restraint protocols. Talk to the person in a nonjudgmental manner and with calm reassurance. This can go a long way toward defusing aggression at an emergency scene until help arrives.

Phencyclidine (PCP)[3]

What is PCP?

PCP is a dissociative anesthetic.

In medicine, PCP (under the trade names Sernyl and Sernylan) was used for anesthesia in the 1950s. Its side effects, however, drove the development of better medications that replaced PCP for clinical use in 1965.

As an illicit drug, PCP is produced in its pure form and in a variety of derivatives. It is a powder or a liquid, and goes by many names: PCP, angel dust, ozone, rocket fuel, wack, trank, and magic dust. It can be snorted, smoked, injected, or taken orally. Users often smoke "dippers," which are cigarettes or marijuana dipped in PCP.

Signs and symptoms of PCP use

- altered awareness
- low blood sugar
- auditory and visual hallucinations
- delusions and paranoia
- violent and/or bizarre behaviors
- euphoria, relaxation, and drowsiness
- panic, terror, and an overwhelming fear of dying
- coma and seizures
- nausea, vomiting, and salivation
- increased heart rate and/or irregular heartbeat (dysrhythmia)
- chills, shivering
- increased body temperature (hyperthermia)
- speech disturbances
- decreased sensitivity to, and awareness of, pain, touch, and position
- painful reaction to sound
- constricted pupils and blurred vision

First-aid alerts for PCP

When PCP is taken with an opioid (or another CNS depressant), it can result in severe respiratory depression or respiratory arrest, which can lead to cardiac arrest and death.

PCP use can cause a significant rise in body temperature (hyperthermia), which can lead to seizures, brain damage, and death if not corrected. Cooling a hyperthermic patient is critically important. Place the person in crisis in the recovery position (provided they are breathing adequately) and pour water on the chest and back. Provide cool cloths.

Selective serotonin reuptake inhibitors (SSRIs)

What are SSRIs?

SSRIs are a family of antidepressant medications. They are the most commonly prescribed antidepressants in North America.

It is believed that SSRIs treat depression by preventing the reuptake (reabsorption) of serotonin, which makes more serotonin available in the brain. Serotonin is a neurotransmitter in the brain, and throughout the body, and is sometimes referred to as the "feel good substance."

SSRIs and opioids in combination can create a potentially fatal condition: serotonin syndrome. This is because SSRIs and opioids *both* prevent the reuptake of serotonin. The result can be dangerously high levels of serotonin in the body. The high levels of serotonin dominate the symptoms of the mixed overdose.

Signs and symptoms of serotonin syndrome

- increased heart rate, pulse strength, and blood pressure
- increased body temperature (hyperthermia)
- increased respiration rate
- tremors (shaking)
- confusion
- sweating
- impaired coordination
- agitation
- dilated pupils

First-aid alerts for serotonin syndrome

Serotonin syndrome can cause a significant rise in body temperature (hyperthermia), which can lead to seizures, brain damage, and death if not corrected. Cooling a hyperthermic patient is critically important. Place the person in crisis in the recovery position (provided they are breathing adequately) and pour water on the chest and back. Provide cool cloths.

The administration of naloxone may be beneficial, because it may temporarily suppress 1 of the stimulants maintaining elevated levels of serotonin.

REFERENCES

1 Substance Abuse and Mental Health Services Administration. Buprenorphine [Internet]. Washington, DC: US Dept of Health and Human Services; 2019 Nov 22 [cited 2020 Feb 4]. Available from https://www.samhsa.gov/medication-assisted-treatment/treatment/buprenorphine

2 Pomara C, Cassano T, D'Errico S, et al. Data available on the extent of cocaine use and dependence: biochemistry, pharmacologic effects and global burden of disease of cocaine abusers. *Curr Med Chem*. 2012;19(33):5647–57.

3 Center for Substance Abuse Research. Phencylidine (PCP) [Internet]. College Park, MD: University of Maryland; 2013 Oct 29 [cited 2020 Feb 18]. Available from http://www.cesar.umd.edu/cesar/drugs/pcp.asp

6

Opioid emergency cases

This chapter recounts opioid emergencies that I have attended as a paramedic with emergency medical services (EMS) or that colleagues have shared with me.

They illustrate the variety of contexts in which opioid emergencies can occur. They also provide concrete examples of rapid response.

Note that follow-up at a hospital is necessary in all cases where naloxone is administered. Opioids remain in the bloodstream longer than naloxone, and their effects can reemerge after a dose of naloxone has worn off. This is why a person in crisis may require several repeat doses of naloxone. In the most severe cases, naloxone can be administered by continuous intravenous (IV) infusion in hospital.

Case 1: Heroin overdose

When I was working as a student paramedic, I completed a rotation in the United States. On several occasions, my team dealt with overdoses, including opioid overdoses and mixed overdoses. One case stands out because of the risks it posed of blood-borne pathogens (in this patient, HIV and hepatitis), and because of the combative response from the patient when I administered naloxone.

This patient was a known IV drug user in a densely populated city in New Jersey. My instructor and I were called to intercept an ambulance with emergency medical technicians (EMTs) on board. At the time of this case, EMTs were not allowed to administer naloxone: it was not in their scope of practice. We got on the ambulance, and were presented with a slim, midthirties female patient with known heroin use, and known HIV and hepatitis risks. The patient was lying in the recovery position on a stretcher with a blanket over her, and was receiving oxygen by mask. She was breathing on her own, but her breathing rate was decreased. The EMTs had placed an oral airway tube in her mouth to support her airway and ventilations. Her pulse was slow and her blood pressure was lower than normal. The team decided to avoid starting an IV line at this time due to the increased risks associated with blood-borne pathogens.

Rapid response

We were all wearing personal protective equipment (PPE). This was one of my first uses of intranasal (IN) naloxone. I drew up 2 mg of naloxone into a 3-mL syringe, removed the needle used to draw up the medication, and replaced it with a luer-lock (screw-on) nasal tip. I then delivered the dose of naloxone up her nostril, and we monitored her for a response. Within a couple minutes, she woke suddenly and aggressively. She was reaching out for things and trying to undo the stretcher straps, and began shouting and complaining about losing her high. We gently restrained her on the stretcher, and tried to calm and reassure her. She became aggressive toward us, angry about us "wasting her high." A team member who had provided care to her in the past was able to calm her down. She remained conscious and calmer for the rest of the 10-minute trip to the hospital, and during the handoff to the emergency hospital team.

What happened?

Opioid addicts can exhibit symptoms of opioid withdrawal on administration of naloxone. These symptoms can include a sudden return of consciousness and sudden aggression. This is a reason to remove potential weapons on or near a person in crisis before you give naloxone.

This case also highlights the advantages of IN naloxone.

Emergency medical services in the US have used IN naloxone since the 1990s, although IN naloxone was barely mentioned in paramedic education in Canada at that time. IN naloxone is now common in EMS in both the

US and Canada, and is especially useful in
ambulances to avoid needlestick injury: starting IV lines and providing needle-based injec-
tions is challenging in a moving ambulance at
the best of times.

Case 2: Unintentional overdose in an EMS procedural sedation

A male in his early twenties reported to our
onsite clinic at a major music event. It was
approximately 11:00 a.m. and he walked in
with his girlfriend. He had a dislocated shoulder—something that had happened to him, he
reported, several times before.

We set him up in a bed, and completed our
initial history and vital signs. He denied any
allergies or medication use, including drugs.
He did say that he had had 1 beer earlier in the
morning, prior to the shoulder injury.

He had regular healthy vital signs, and was
very conscious and alert. Our team decided
to give him medications to provide pain relief
and sedation before arranging transport to the
local hospital, which involved a 20-minute trip
by ambulance.

With the assistance of 2 EMT students, I
placed an IV line, and began to administer
fluids and sedation with midazolam, a benzodiazepine. After monitoring him for several
minutes, I administered IV fentanyl, in small
amounts, while continuing to monitor his
response and pain levels. I was attempting to
reduce his pain so we could sling and swathe
his dislocated shoulder, and hand him off to

an EMS ambulance crew. In the course of 5 to 10 minutes, I repeated the IV fentanyl in small amounts.

After 15 minutes and several small-dose IV administrations of fentanyl, he became relaxed. When asked if we could sling and swathe his shoulder, he agreed. During the moments the team prepared the bandaging, he slumped back on the bed and lost consciousness. I attempted to rouse him with verbal and painful stimulus, but he remained unresponsive. After several moments, he stopped breathing spontaneously (apnea).

Rapid response

I immediately laid him back, tilted his neck, and opened his mouth to maintain his airway. I had my EMT team members provide bag-valve-mask ventilations with oxygen attached.

I then immediately prepared a 2.0-mg dose of naloxone by manual draw, and pushed the dose into the IV line over 30 to 60 seconds. Within minutes of administering the naloxone, he regained consciousness and resumed normal breathing.

Note that my team and I had already put on gloves to care for this patient's injury. The team members operating the bag valve mask added safety glasses to their PPE to minimize the risk of contact with droplets or possible vomitus. This was enough PPE for the overdose that arose: in this monitored setting, the overdose posed no unknown risks of opioid exposure.

What happened?

After we delved into his history in more detail, he and his girlfriend admitted that he had had 11 beers that morning—not the single beer he had reported. The pain of the shoulder dislocation had made him appear more sober than he actually was. The administration of the benzodiazepine and fentanyl would have been fine if he had been sober, but they caused unconsciousness when mixed with the depressant effects of the alcohol. We monitored him until it was safe to transport him to hospital. He returned later in the day to thank us for the care.

As a relatively new paramedic to sedation (at that time), I learned very quickly the effects of fentanyl and its potency, particularly in the presence of other drugs, alcohol, and medications. I have now assisted and completed more than 200 procedural sedations, and, to this day, have never had a recurrence of this event. Even to trained health-care providers, the effects of opioids and the risk of overdose are ever present. Naloxone and all emergency resuscitation gear are mandatory for all health-care providers when giving opioids.

Case 3: Unintentional overdose in a clinical setting

A 20-year-old male came to his dentist for IV sedation for the removal of wisdom teeth.

Before we discuss this case, let's quickly look at a common method of procedural sedation for dental patients. Once a patient has undergone health-care screening, assessment of vital signs, and questions about their medical and medication history, a plan for sedation is created. The patient is provided with an IV line and often receives 2 medications separately to induce sedation, relaxation, and amnesia. This 2-drug technique often involves a benzodiazepine known as midazolam (Versed), and fentanyl, which increases the effectiveness of midazolam. Both drugs act to depress the central nervous system, so patients have a number of monitors attached to them, such as a cardiac monitor (ECG), pulse oximeter (this reads oxygen levels in blood), blood-pressure monitor, and respiration monitor. Some facilities also monitor carbon dioxide and other important signs to ensure safety.

The patient in this case was healthy, had no medical conditions, and denied taking any medications prior to the procedure.

The dentist and 2 other health-care staff attended the sedation procedure. As the team prepared the IV line and the medications, they reconfirmed the patient's history. They then provided the patient with the benzodiazepine slowly by IV injection. Within several minutes, they provided a small dose of IV fentanyl. The health-care team monitored the patient closely. Within 2 minutes, the patient stopped breathing.

The team tried to wake him with verbal and painful stimulus. He did not respond. He was unconscious and unresponsive. He had a strong pulse at this time.

Rapid response

The dentist directed the 2 other health-care staff to provide ventilations via bag valve mask with oxygen attached. Within 10 to 15 seconds, the team members opened the airway by tilting the head back and elevating the lower jaw (mandible). At this time, the dentist reached for an ampoule of naloxone and quickly provided 2 mg of naloxone in the IV line. The patient regained consciousness and normal breathing within 2 minutes. The team called EMS (911), which responded to the scene.

Note that the health-care staff already had on PPE for the dental procedure (masks, gowns, gloves, and eye protection) and did not need more PPE for the overdose crisis. The overdose in this monitored setting posed no unknown risks of opioid exposure.

What happened?

The patient later said he had taken three Tylenol 3 pills approximately 1 hour prior to his appointment. He did not inform the health-care team, although asked twice about medication use. He stated that he received the Tylenol 3 from a friend, who said it would be helpful to control the pain of wisdom-tooth extraction. He did not want to tell the dentist or the team what he had done.

Tylenol 3 contains 30 mg of codeine (an opioid) per pill. In combination with the fentanyl and midazolam, it was enough opioid to produce respiratory arrest. Even though the health-care team did everything correctly, this incident occurred. Thankfully it occurred with a trained and prepared team.

In all cases of procedural sedation, health-care providers have naloxone available for opioid overdose, and a reversal medication called flumazenil for benzodiazepine overdose. This reversal preparation is mandatory for most procedural sedation in health-care settings.

Case 4: Overdose at a concert

A 19-year-old female was attending a concert. She had been drinking for a few hours and smoking marijuana with friends. At the concert, she and her friends opened a new bag of marijuana, which they had purchased illegally. Several moments after smoking this marijuana, the female lost consciousness and went into respiratory arrest.

Rapid response

I was a member of the special-event EMS team at the concert that responded.

When we arrived, she was on her back with a friend close by. Her friend reported that she had "passed out" and was not breathing properly.

The team put on full PPE and then assessed her. The team found:

- She was unconscious and unresponsive to verbal and painful stimulus.

- She was not breathing on her own (no spontaneous ventilations).

- Her pulse was slow and regular at the neck (carotid artery). The team also checked her wrist (radial artery) and did not feel a pulse.

We opened her airway, quickly suctioning it of saliva. We gave her artificial ventilations with a bag valve mask that was attached to oxygen. We determined that she had a significant risk of opioid overdose. We gave her a 4-mg dose of nasal naloxone, and continued bag-valve-mask ventilations. Within 2 minutes, she opened her eyes. She remained conscious for approximately 30 seconds, and then quickly went unconscious again and stopped breathing. The team continued bag-valve-mask ventilations and provided a second 4-mg dose of nasal naloxone. Within 1 to 2 minutes, she completely regained consciousness and began breathing on her own (spontaneous ventilations).

We completed a head-to-toe survey looking for injuries or other causes of medical crisis, and established an IV line. We then handed the patient over to an ambulance EMS team for care and transport to hospital.

What happened?

In review of the case by speaking with the patient and the friend, health-care providers determined that the female was the only one to smoke the illegally purchased marijuana. They concluded that this marijuana had been laced with fentanyl.

Fentanyl can be mixed into almost any substance. It is common to find fentanyl mixed in street drugs such as marijuana, methamphetamine, cocaine, heroin pills, and fake pills resembling oxycodone.

7

A primer on opioids, opioid use, and addiction

In North America, opioid overdoses and deaths from overdoses are at epidemic levels. Each year, 75,000 to 100,000 lives are lost to opioid overdoses in Canada and the United States.

The great majority of these deaths are due to fentanyl, a synthetic opioid medication created in 1959.

Many are also due to carfentanil, another synthetic opioid.

Opiates versus opioids

Opiates are compounds naturally derived from the sap of the opium poppy.[1] Opium poppies grow wild and are cultivated in many parts of the world. The sap leaks from mature

opium poppies, and is then scraped from the
plants and dried. The dried extract forms the
base ingredient of opium.

Opioids are semisynthetic or completely
synthetic compounds that produce opium-like
effects, or that bind to opioid receptors in the
body.[1]

Semisynthetic opioids

Semisynthetic opioids are created by chemi-
cally modifying opiates.

They are used in some over-the-counter
medications in some jurisdictions (e.g.,
codeine), in prescription medications (e.g.,
codeine, morphine), and in illicit drugs
(e.g., heroin).

Synthetic opioids

Synthetic opioids are manufactured without
opiates.

Synthetic opioids are used as prescription
medications, in veterinary medicine, and in
illicit drugs.

Starting in 2013, death rates from the illegal use of synthetic opioids, including fentanyl
and others, began to significantly increase
in North America. Synthetic opioids were
discovered in the twentieth century and were
approved for use in medicine as follows:

Fentanyl	1964
Carfentanil	1974 (veterinary use only)
Sufentanil	1980
Alfentanil	1984
Remifentanil	1999

The United Nations Office on Drugs and Crime (UNODC) documents that 17 fentanyl analogues were reported between 2012 and 2016.[2(p4)] A fentanyl analogue is a chemical derivative or modification of fentanyl.

Medications that contain opiates and opioids

Opioids are primarily used for cough suppression, diarrhea control, pain management (including chronic pain), and to aid in the sedation of patients undergoing medical, dental, orthopedic, and other medical procedures.

Codeine is the least potent type of opioid. It is used for pain management and cough suppression, and is available over the counter in many jurisdictions. Tylenol 1, 2, 3, and 4 all contain codeine along with their base ingredient of acetaminophen. In many jurisdictions, Tylenol 1 can be purchased without a prescription (over the counter). It includes 8 mg of codeine. Tylenol 2, 3, and 4 require a prescription and have 15 mg, 30 mg, and 60 mg of codeine respectively.

When these medications do not meet the pain-control needs of a patient, stronger medications may be prescribed. Pain management can become an issue for patients with chronic pain, or pain due to potentially terminal diseases such as cancer. Stronger opioid-based pain medications include OxyContin, Vicodin, and Percocet.

Morphine and **fentanyl** may also be prescribed when doctors feel stronger

opioid-based pain medications are needed.
Fentanyl is available in pill form, lozenge, and
in transdermal patches applied to the skin to
absorb over time. Some cancer and palliative
patients are prescribed injectable morphine
by their physician for use at home, or within
a palliative care center in the community.
These legal sources of opioids are both helpful
and therapeutic when patients are in close
communication with their physicians about
their specific pain needs. Advanced care paramedics, nurse practitioners, and physician
assistants working in the community also have
access to these medications, which are safe
and effective when administered by a health-
care professional.

Comparing opioids

Opioids fall on a spectrum of potency. Let's
assign morphine a potency of 1. The spectrum
then looks like this:

Morphine	1
Oxycodone	1 to 2
Methadone	3 to 7
Hydromorphone	5
Buprenorphine	40
Heroin	50
Fentanyl	50 to 100
Sufentanil	500 to 1,000
Carfentanil	10,000 to 100,000

Carfentanil was designed for large mam-
mals in veterinary care. It is not designed for

humans, due to its intense concentration. Exposure to even minute amounts of carfentanil can cause overdose or death in humans.

What do opioids do in the body?

In addition to their beneficial actions of pain management and controlled sedation, opioids have other effects that are not desired.

All opioids, once they enter the body, ultimately find their way into the bloodstream. In an opioid emergency, this is why the route of exposure is important. If the drug is injected directly into the bloodstream, it will have the quickest onset of action. For drug users, this can result in situations where they die with the needle still in their arm.

Once in the bloodstream, opioids attach to opioid receptors. A receptor in the body is like a lock waiting for the right key. Once the right key enters the lock, the receptor activates. This causes a reaction to occur in the body.

In our body, we have different types of opioid receptors, in different locations and tissues.

For example, opioid receptors exist in our digestive system, particularly our large intestine. Once opioids attach in this location, they slow the function of the bowel considerably, causing constipation. This is why if you've ever been on codeine for pain control, or loperamide for diarrhea control, you may have experienced constipation. Some common antidiarrhea medications are designed to mimic this opioid-intestine effect. They attach

to the receptors in the large intestine and slow
bowel function, preventing or reducing the
risk of diarrhea.

Other opioid receptors can have more
dangerous consequences. Opioids that attach
to the respiratory centers of the nervous system can slow breathing or stop it completely,
depending on the amount of opioid. This is
why codeine is a powerful cough suppres-
sant (antitussive). Codeine also, for the same
reason, increases vulnerability to airway
obstruction. Any drug that diminishes your
cough reflex makes you vulnerable to airway
problems.

When a person overdoses on a drug con-
taining opioids, the biggest risk is to breathing, which will at least slow and may stop.
A person who stops breathing is in respiratory
arrest. If not corrected, by a rescuer opening
the airway and delivering ventilations, the
victim will progress deeper into shock, and
ultimately cardiac arrest will occur. We cannot
live long without adequate respirations.

Why do people become addicted to opioids?

Pain control and addiction

For many users of opioids in medical circumstances, and under the careful eye of their
health-care providers, opioids are helpful and
beneficial. However, a number of people with
pain and chronic pain due to injury and disease become addicted to opioids.

Any substance or activity has the potential for addiction. Addiction is "a compulsive, chronic, physiological or psychological need for a habit-forming substance, behavior, or activity having harmful physical, psychological, or social effects and typically causing well-defined symptoms (such as anxiety, irritability, tremors, or nausea) upon withdrawal or abstinence."[3]

Many people who are prescribed opioids don't become addicted. They may have prescriptions for opioids after release from a health-care facility, as they heal from an injury, surgical procedure, or disease. Most patients finish the prescribed medication and stop without a problem. Or they may stop before the prescribed medication runs out, because their pain decreases or because they don't like the side effects of opioids (e.g., constipation, nausea, euphoria).

A percentage of patients who have received opioid-containing pain medications, however, become addicted. Opioids are highly addictive in certain individuals, and prescribed pain-control medication is a common route to addiction. When these patients can no longer access prescription pain control, they often seek illicit sources of opioids. People who have been on prescription opioids for pain are more likely to become addicted to stronger drugs.

People become addicted to other drugs, too, and may end up in an opioid emergency through use of these drugs. Addiction can occur because of mental-health or other challenges with complex origins.

The person you assist in an opioid crisis could easily be a neighbor, a family member, a coworker, or anyone from anywhere and any walk of life. Addiction crosses all socioeconomic boundaries. As a member of society, and when providing first aid, it is essential not to judge the person you are assisting.

Patients with chronic pain, patients with cancer, and patients with pain in palliative care require constant long-term pain control. For physicians and researchers that specialize in chronic pain management, this is a challenge. Research continues into nonopioid medications and alternative therapies for chronic pain.

Stories of addiction and overdose

In my work as a paramedic and in teaching first aid, cardiopulmonary resuscitation (CPR), and programs in prehospital care, a number of students and health-care providers have shared stories of opioid dependence with me. They are very personal stories of injury, trauma, mental and physical pain, and addiction.

One person had injured his back in the workplace. A physician evaluated the injury and prescribed a pain-relieving medication that contained codeine. He completed his medication after 2 weeks, and also completed physiotherapy. He said he still felt pain after this, but admitted he noticed improvement. He went back to his physician and got an extension of the medication for another 2 to 4 weeks, as needed. This began his addiction to prescription opioids. He took them for more than 20 years.

When I asked why, he described the reduction in pain, the sensation of euphoria, and the feeling of the high of the opioid. He said the actual pain of the back injury had subsided years earlier, but he continued to report pain during physical exams and visits to his physician. Essentially, he learned how to manipulate the system and to lie to his physician to feed his addiction.

After trying on several occasions to stop using opioids, he finally succeeded. Thankfully this was a success story: this person was able to wean himself off opioids. Not every story ends like this, unfortunately.

In another story, a student let me know that a family member, recently diagnosed with terminal cancer, had been prescribed strong opioid medications for pain control. This included fentanyl in the form of transdermal patches worn on the skin, which allow the drug to absorb slowly. It also included oxycodone pills. After several weeks of using these medications, the family member was found in cardiac arrest. Other family members began CPR and contacted emergency medical services for assistance. It was later confirmed that the patient had overdosed on opioids. It was not determined whether this was an intentional or accidental overdose.

Addiction and withdrawal

When a person is addicted to opioids, they must have the opioid to cope with daily life.

Without the opioid, they go into withdrawal.
The signs and symptoms of opioid withdrawal
can be severe and potentially life-threatening.
They may include chills, goose bumps, rapid
heart rate, rapid breathing, tremors, nervous-
ness, aggressive behavior, and seizures. When
you consider addiction, it's important to realize that an addicted person might die without
the substance they are addicted to. This is why
the management and care of a person undergoing detoxification must occur in a medical
facility.

The duration of withdrawal and rehabilitation can take from 5 days to several weeks.
Methadone (another form of opioid) and
buprenorphine-naloxone are often used to aid
in rehabilitation under medical supervision.

Rehabilitation programs vary greatly from
region to region. Social and medical programs
for detoxification and rehabilitation from
alcohol and drug dependency have existed for
many years. The escalating opioid crisis has
overwhelmed many rehabilitation centers.

Naloxone and withdrawal

Naloxone, provided to an addicted and overdosed person, provokes some or all of the
signs and symptoms of withdrawal.

Naloxone does not provoke these symptoms in an overdosed person who is not
addicted to opioids. Consider a situation
where a friend, family member, or emergency
worker, who is not an opioid user, unknow-
ingly encounters fentanyl or carfentanil powder. The exposure may be significant enough

to cause overdose or cardiac arrest. If you were able to safely provide first aid and deliver naloxone to this person, they might show confusion or agitation after resuscitation, but they would not show signs or symptoms of withdrawal.

Here's another situation: a person takes too many prescribed painkillers with codeine. Perhaps the person is seeking more pain relief than the prescription can deliver, if taken as directed, or perhaps they misread the label. In either case, the person may overdose, although not addicted to opioids. If given naloxone, they would not show signs or symptoms of withdrawal.

The role of fentanyl and carfentanil in overdosing

For drug dealers and traffickers, fentanyl and carfentanil can increase the potency, duration of effect, and addictive properties of the illegal drugs they sell. These synthetic opioids are easy to buy or to make in clandestine (illegal) labs, and they can be mixed with a variety of other street drugs.

The majority of illegal fentanyl in the world currently comes from China, but this may change. Clandestine labs for synthetic opioids now operate in many parts of North America, similar to meth labs. Compared to methamphetamine, synthetic opioids (including fentanyl, fentanyl analogues, and carfentanil) are simpler to produce from a chemistry standpoint. In addition, according to UNODC, the

equipment needed to produce synthetic opioids is easily accessible.[2(p7)]

Drug dealers and traffickers mix illegal
fentanyl into heroin, marijuana, methamphetamine, cocaine, and other drugs. They also
make fentanyl into pills, or add fentanyl to
fake pills that look like pharmaceutical-grade
opioid medications.

People purchasing fake pills often believe
they are purchasing pharmaceutical-grade
pills for their addiction. Pharmaceutical-grade
pills may also be for sale illegally; these have
been stolen or diverted from the legitimate
chain of supply. It is hard for users to know
what is real and what is fake. Fake pills closely
resemble OxyContin, Percocet, and Vicodin,
and they may be laced with fentanyl, and, in
some cases, carfentanil. People using fake pills
can become overdosed because of added synthetic opioids.

Some drug users know that they are purchasing pure fentanyl pills, which they seek
as their addiction needs become stronger.
Heroin users often turn to fentanyl to get a
more intense high. It is easier to overdose on
fentanyl than heroin, due to its potency.

People who use recreational drugs, or who
are addicted to street drugs, can overdose
on what they believe to be marijuana, methamphetamine, or cocaine, unaware of added
synthetic opioids.

At some safe-injection sites, addicts can
have street drugs tested for synthetic opioids.
Sadly, some addicts choose to use drugs with
fentanyl or carfentanil anyway, because of the

strength of their addiction. In some jurisdictions, safe-injection sites are considered controversial, but they provide a way to address the increasing problem of opioid addiction through harm reduction. They provide judgment-free areas for addicts to access shelter, clean needles and syringes, and health-care-provider oversight in the event of an overdose.

Another harm-reduction initiative, the MySafe project, uses vending machines to provide prescribed amounts of hydromorphone to opioid addicts. The machines provide addicts with judgment-free access to pharmaceutical-grade drugs free of synthetic opioids. The first MySafe vending machine was installed in Vancouver in February 2020.[4]

REFERENCES

1 Nelson LS, Hoffman RS, Howland MA, Lewin NA, Goldfrank LR, Smith SW. *Goldfrank's Toxicologic Emergencies.* 11th ed. New York: McGraw-Hill Education; 2019. 2096 p.

2 United Nations Office on Drugs and Crime. Fentanyl and its analogues—50 years on. Vienna: United Nations Office on Drugs and Crime, Global SMART programme; 2017 March. 12 p. (Global SMART update series; vol. 17).

3 Meriiam-Webster.com [Internet]. [Springfield, MA]: Merriam-Webster.com; 2020 [cited 2020 Jan 24]. Available from https://www.merriam-webster.com/dictionary/addiction

4 Opioid vending machine opens in Vancouver: MySafe scheme for addicts aims to help reduce opioid deaths in Canadian city. *The Guardian* [Internet]; 2020 Feb 17 [cited 2020 Feb 19]. Available from https://www.theguardian.com/science/2020/feb/17/opioid-vending-machine-opens-vancouver-mysafe-canada

Abbreviations

ABCs	airway, breathing, circulation
AED	automatic external defibrillator
BAC	blood-alcohol concentration
BBFE	blood and body fluid exposure
CNS	central nervous system
CPR	cardiopulmonary resuscitation
CSA	Canadian Standards Association (CSA Group)
ECG	electrocardiogram
EMS	emergency medical services
EMT	emergency medical technician
ER	emergency room
GHB	gamma-hydroxybutyrate
IM	intramuscular
IN	intranasal
IV	intravenous
LOC	level of consciousness
LSD	lysergic acid diethylamide
MDMA	3,4-methylenedioxymethamphetamine (ecstasy)
NIOSH	National Institute for Occupational Safety and Health
PCP	phencyclidine
PFAK	personal first-aid kit
PPE	personal protective equipment
SCA	sudden cardiac arrest
SCBA	self-contained breathing apparatus
SSRI	selective serotonin reuptake inhibitor
THC	tetrahydrocannabinol
UNODC	United Nations Office on Drugs and Crime

Free download

Always be ready to deal with an opioid emergency wherever you are. Download and print out this handy wallet-sized card with simple, step-by-step instructions at **brusheducation.ca/opioids**

To assist a person in crisis

1. Assess level of consciousness.
2. If unresponsive, open the airway.
3. Clear the mouth.
4. Assess breathing and pulse.
5. No pulse: start CPR
   (30 chest compressions per 2 ventilations, or 30:2).
6. Pulse, but inadequate breathing: start rescue ventilations (1 per 5 to 6 seconds).
7. Administer naloxone.
8. Administer more naloxone as needed.
9. Continued unconsciousness: rule out other reasons.
10. Watch for symptoms of mixed overdose.

Want to learn more and build your skills?

Check out Greg Clarkes's online training for opioid emergencies, complete with videos and quizzes.

Visit RapidResponseGuides.com to register.

About the author

Greg Clarkes, ACP, NRP, is an advanced care paramedic registered in Canada and the United States. He is a clinic-based paramedic for Primco Dene EMS at Cenovus Energy's oil sands project on the Cold Lake Air Weapons Range in Alberta, Canada. He also works in dentistry as a sedation monitoring assistant. Greg has more than 30 years' experience as an educator in emergency medical services, and has spoken and taught internationally throughout his career. He founded the Canadian First Aid School in 1988 and the Canadian College of EMS in 1996. He serves as the education coordinator at the school and college, where he teaches basic and advanced life support, tactical combat casualty care, and emergency care in dental sedation. He has served as an executive committee member of the Advanced Medical Life Support program with National Association of Emergency Medical Technicians (NAEMT) in the US, as its only international member. He volunteered for 15 years as the Canadian coordinator with NAEMT, in its Prehospital Trauma Life Support (PHTLS), Advanced Medical Life Support (AMLS), and Emergency Pediatric Care (EPC) programs. Greg has served in the naval reserve, and worked in security and private investigation.